PRAISE
WHAT'S MY BODY

Dr. Anthea's book gives you a wor̄___ ___ __ __ __ __
work out what is going on with your body, what your body is telling you,
and how to listen to it. Then she gives you a pathway back to health.
She is the voice you have been looking for, with knowledge, expertise,
intuition, and an unbelievable ability to make things that seem
impossibly hard to understand simple and easy to "just get!"
—Dr. Annette Colman, DC

Dr. Anthea is a brilliant, playful, and kind friend to all women.
She delivers her sage advice with intelligence and comedy, candid
but never patronizing. Whatever that magic is, I am glad she has it.
—Tiffani Clingin, BSW, GCFT, GCTRP, MAPP

In What's My Body Telling Me?, *Dr. Anthea delves into the*
intricate world of women's health with a fresh and innovative perspective.
Dr. Anthea navigates the complexities of the female body, offering a holistic
approach that goes beyond conventional methods. This book seamlessly
blends scientific insight with practical advice, empowering readers to
understand and optimize their wellbeing. With a focus on holistic
wellness, this work emerges as an indispensable guide for those
seeking a transformative journey toward balanced and vibrant health.
—Dr. Sarah Jane Perri, DC, Spinal Energetics

Dr. Anthea takes what could be confusing, stressful, or frustrating
and packages it up clearly and easily. This book has the answers that you've
been searching for, and Anthea delivers them with her amazing combination
of humor, intelligence, and empathy. You'll leave this book with a renewed
faith in your own body and some clear steps on what's next.
—Dr. Virginia Croke, DC

What's My Body Telling Me?

What's My Body Telling Me?

YOUR BODY ISN'T THE PROBLEM. IT'S THE SOLUTION.

Dr. Anthea Todd
Founder of Female Fundamentals™

First published in 2024 by Dean Publishing
PO Box 119
Mt. Macedon, Victoria, 3441
Australia
deanpublishing.com

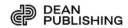

DEAN PUBLISHING

Cataloguing-in-Publication Data
National Library of Australia

Title: What's My Body Telling Me?
ISBN: 978-1-925452-81-5
Category: Women's health

The views and opinions expressed in this book are those of the author and do not necessarily reflect the official policy or position of any other agency, publisher, organization, employer, medical body or company. Assumptions made in the analysis are not reflective of the position of any entity other than the author(s) — and, these views are always subject to change, revision, and rethinking at any time.

The author, publisher or organizations are not to be held responsible for misuse, reuse, recycled and cited and/or uncited copies of content within this book by others.

This book is educational only and not intended as a substitute for the medical advice of physicians. The reader should regularly consult a trusted physician in matters relating to their personal health, particularly with respect to any symptoms that may require diagnosis or medical attention. The ideas within this book are only the opinion of the author and are not intended to replace any medical advice or diagnose or treat any health issues.

Although health issues are discussed in the book, it is advised to not use this book as an alternative or substitute for medical treatment. Individuals are advised to always take their health matters into their own hands.

Please note: When discussing women's health, the author is utilising her knowledge of the female XX genotype and its specific role in female health. Throughout the book the words female and woman/women are used interchangeably for readability however the author recognizes one refers to gender and the other sex.

Names, occupations, ages, and personal health issues depicted within the publication have been changed to protect the identity of individuals.

DEDICATION

**To any woman who has ever felt
that her body was the problem.**

Dr. Anthea shares free resources
and additional support links
at the back of this book.

You can also grab your
exclusive book bonuses here:
www.femalefundamentals.com.au/book-bonuses

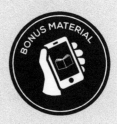

Contents

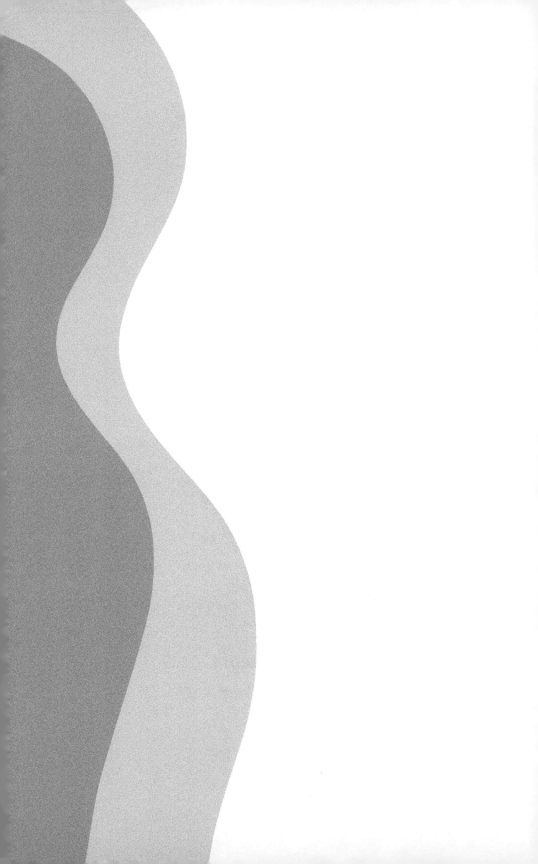

Introduction

HOW I GOT HERE

~

Mum always said, "Never go straight for the clitoris..."

My mum is a chiropractor and when training new practitioners, she advises them not to rush in and tell people what's wrong without listening to them first. She believes in warming up the environment before diving into a clinical diagnosis. She phrases it as, "Never go straight for the clitoris." I guess that's good advice in general.

I believe she originally stole the line from a Monty Python skit but used it among chiropractors to promote awareness and mindfulness (and possibly provide some useful sex advice). It also highlights her optimism—she was clearly confident that a good portion of her trainees could locate the clitoris first go.

I was thirteen years old when I first understood the importance of medicine.

One sunny Sunday morning at the beach, I was training for Nippers, which is like surf lifesaving for kids. Mum happened to be my age group's coordinator for the morning, and we'd been tasked with doing three back-to-back Ironman circuits. For those who don't know, an Ironman circuit consists of running 200 m, swimming 200 m around floating cans in the ocean, running again, and then paddling a board around those same cans. We did that three times without a break! It seems my mum either had a death wish for us or she just didn't understand how hard it would be.

After completing my second round of the Ironman circuit, I was running into the water for the final swim when my legs started to collapse underneath me. Thankfully, I was only ankle-deep. I thought to myself, *If I try to swim, I'm going to drown.* So, I turned around and staggered my way back up the beach. Mum was hollering, "Keep going, Anthea"—but I couldn't. I could barely speak. (Side note: one thing you should also know about me is I'm competitive. I don't like to give up and if I'm doing something, I'm trying my hardest to win. Thankfully, I listened to my body and not my head that day). When I almost passed out right there on the sand, Mum realized how exhausted I was.

She told me to lie down and breathe. After five minutes of me breathing heavily, she took my pulse: 210 beats per minute. For those playing at home, the max your heart rate should be is 220 minus your age. So, technically, I was still at my max heart rate after five minutes rest.

Fast-forward another ten minutes, and it had only gone down to 200 beats. As luck would have it, the local pediatrician also had kids doing Nippers, so Mum called him over to the first-aid tower. He took my pulse and after forty-five minutes of rest, it was still 175 beats per minute, which, in summary, is *no bueno*. Something was wrong. We needed to find out what was happening inside my body.

After several months of investigations, six-hour round trips to Melbourne, seven days of Holter monitors with wires and sticky patches, we found that I had a hole in my heart. It's what they call an atrial septal defect, where the oxygenated blood mixes with the deoxygenated blood, making my heart work extra hard for the same result. Plus, I had some extra centers in my heart that caused it to beat really fast when it wasn't meant to. As my cardiologist said, I needed a heart plumber and a heart electrician. Greedy!

Being only thirteen years old, it was the most I had been in a hospital and around traditional medical practices. In fact, prior to my heart condition, I had never really thought of medicine as a necessary part of life.

Coming from a lineage of chiropractors, I was raised with the mindset: *if something's wrong, your body is telling you something.* This was normal in our family. It took me some time to realize that this mindset isn't everyone's "normal"—far from it. Or maybe my family is just weird. We considered the human body to be the best doctor. To us, medicine was available when our bodies needed that kind of support, but it wasn't the main character of the show; it was an extra. Kinda like Rebel Wilson in *Bridesmaids*, not the main character but the best supporting cameo.

I was in high school when I first started to recognize that the perspective I had on health was different from most people's. When I had a headache, I wouldn't ask my friends if they had a Panadol in their school bags, unlike most of my friends. Instead, I figured I either needed more water, needed to take a break from the noise and commotion and breathe, or I hadn't had enough sleep. When I had period pain, I considered how to function with it and questioned what I had been doing in the months leading up to it that could be affecting it. Then on the rare occasion when I couldn't function, I would be home with a hot water bottle and rest, or, in dire circumstances, I would have an anti-inflammatory so I could still do what I needed to do. Viewing something as simple as a headache or period pain as a sign that my body was talking to me was just the norm. No matter the symptom, I was raised to look for the reason behind it.

Within my family, the help we reached for depended on the severity of the problem and the circumstances on the day. We never ran from or avoided the physiological messages of our bodies. We saw our bodies as full wise systems rather than separate parts, and we listened to the messages they gave. I guess that's why Mum's clitoris advice was actually about listening first.

Now, you might be thinking, *Why wouldn't you just take the fucking pain relief?* This is the twenty-first century, and we have medication for a reason. In order to understand how I got here, you need to understand a little more about where I came from.

MINI MEDICINE WOMAN

When I was in grade two, we were given homework. The idea was to pick a theme, like animals or plants, find words in the dictionary, and learn to spell and understand them.

I decided my theme would be the human body. Mum was busy with five kids, as my little sister Claudia was just born, so she told me to wait for Dad to get home and do the homework with him.

Now, you'd think teaching an eight-year-old about the body would consist of things like arm, brain, leg, skin. But no, not *my* dad. We went deep, talking about the hippocampus, a part of the brain that's important for memory. The hypothalamus, sternocleidomastoid, and glomerulus. If you're thinking these words seem like absolute gibberish, then your face may resemble that of my teacher, Mrs. Dalgleish, when I arrived at school the next day and presented her with my homework.

My healthy obsession with the human body helped me persuade my parents to let me stay up past my bedtime on Thursday nights to watch *ER* and then *Grey's Anatomy.* We'd compete to guess the diagnosis of the patient first.

We'd also play games on long family car trips, like the "body part game." One of us would say a body part, and the next person would have to say one that started with the letter that the previous one ended with. For example, if I said "liver," the person after me would say something starting with R, like "rectum." Whenever my turn came after my little brother, Jeremy, I knew I'd need a body part starting with K because you can probably imagine an eight-year-old's favorite phallic body part to scream in the car, knowing he won't get in trouble.

As we got older, our people-watching skills were put into overdrive. We would drive past people walking on the street, and Mum and Dad would say things like, "See how that person is walking? They need a hip replacement on the right. Or they've had a stroke on the left. Or they have a nerve root lesion at L5. We know this because…" This was the norm for us. Some families watch sport together and know how teams should change their tactics. Other families understand music and how a piece of music is arranged. We learned the art of understanding the body.

For my entire life, most of my family have been involved in healthcare to some degree. Both of my parents are chiropractors, the type who seriously love what they do, the type who sees what they do as potentially life-changing for their patients. Several of my aunties, uncles, and cousins (on both sides) are chiropractors too. My grandma was a naturopath, and two of my siblings are also chiropractors. (I did warn you we're kinda weird). Some of our closest family friends are local GPs and surgeons, so healthcare has been an obvious theme throughout my life.

Can you imagine the type of dinner conversations I grew up around? It often consisted of Mum and Dad troubleshooting difficult patient cases and making fun games for us to play along and test our knowledge. Dad might say, "Okay everyone… I'm a thirty-seven-year-old woman with persistent fatigue and heavy periods. What investigations do we need to do? And what is the most likely cause connecting these symptoms?" When other families were playing Monopoly, we were playing "guess the ambiguous medical issue." Fun for the whole family, right?

We would always speak in a way that highlighted how miraculous the body is and the extraordinary things it does. I also got to experience this firsthand when, one day, I ended up in the Melbourne hospital, covered in sand, wearing nothing but a rashie, bather bottoms, zinc on my face, and given a totally different outlook on life.

It was a couple of months after my third and final heart surgery. Everything with my heart was A-OK, and I was back at the same beach where I'd first realized something was wrong. I was now two years older and doing my bronze medallion camp. All was well, but something or someone must have felt like I needed another message about just how precious life is and how important medicine can be…

We were out having fun catching waves on the rescue boards. I caught a wave at the same time as one of the guys in the camp. We both came off, and little did we know that his 11 kg rescue board was still in the air. Just as the tide went out, my feet touched the bottom of the ocean floor, and, at the same time, the board came crashing down onto my head, compressing my spine. (You may be thinking, *Luckily, you have chiropractic parents!*). The weird thing was, I didn't feel any pain in my head. It was instant shooting pain down my neck and into my arms that I felt. Again luckily, my older sister, Morgan, was running the camp for the week and was on the beach, watching the whole thing unfold. She got me to sit down on the sand and eventually stabilized my neck and got me walking up to the clubhouse. She called Mum and explained what happened. Mum left our home, which was twenty minutes away, to come and check me over. Before hanging up, she said, "If anything changes, call me back."

As soon as she hung up, I started to get tingling sensations in my hands and feet, which I now know isn't good. A phone call and an unflattering neck brace later, Mum was there in what felt like less than five minutes (but for legal reasons, let's just say it was twenty). After a quick neurological assessment of my spinal cord, brain, and nerves, Mum was on the phone to the ambulance. I remember saying to her that everything was fine and I didn't want an ambulance, but, based on my symptoms, the dispatcher decided that a helicopter ride to Melbourne was needed. So, dazed, half in and out of consciousness, riding a chopper, I arrived with Mum at the Royal Children's Hospital, three hours' drive from home.

I was rushed into one of the trauma bays with around eight different doctors and nurses poking, prodding, shining lights, and asking me questions. Based on the results, they needed to do an MRI to confirm the cause of my symptoms. It was clear from my assessments that I had pressure on my spinal cord, but it could have been for multiple reasons. The worst could have been a spinal fracture, meaning probable surgery and possible permanent damage to my spinal cord, affecting my ability to control my bodily functions below the neck. Or it could have been swelling, causing something called "spinal shock," that was pressing on the spinal cord, causing the same symptoms, but the effects would pass.

The nine hours I spent lying flat on my back, unable to move, caused me to reflect on how precious life really is. How it could change in an instant. How much I took for granted. How my body just worked: it did everything I needed and wanted it to do, without me consciously needing to ask it. How I could sit up and feed myself without a second thought. How if I needed to go to the toilet, I could just get up and walk there without a bedpan or a catheter. How I could run and use my legs (even though I hated running). How I could play in the surf with my friends. How I could effortlessly do whatever I wanted with my body without a second thought. Those nine hours felt like nine days.

Thankfully, the MRI showed I had spinal swelling caused by a perfect storm of physical trauma to the spine plus the blood thinners I was on after having heart surgery, which made my body and spinal cord more susceptible to inflammation.

I was given the all clear by the doctors, leaving me stranded in a Melbourne hospital in nothing but my bather bottoms and a rashie, with zinc on my face. But my body was fully intact, and I felt deep gratitude for the medical system and the professionals who came to my aid. My soul was so grateful for the life and body I had. Plus I was stoked that one of the nurses gave me a spare set of scrubs pants to wear home, making me feel like I was on the set of *Grey's Anatomy.*

A NEW WAVE OF HEALTHCARE

The culmination of all of these life experiences led to me wanting to study either medicine or chiropractic by the time high school ended. Ultimately, chiropractic won out and after five years of study, I was out in the "real world," able to finally put all of my knowledge and life experience to good use.

When I first began working as a chiropractor, I was in my element, helping people with their symptoms and teaching them about the power of their bodies. Sometimes, I would need to refer patients to medical practitioners to investigate potentially worrisome conditions. Often, they would return in bewilderment and say, "They said there was nothing wrong with me," or, "They said my problem is just part of being a woman."

It didn't take long before I realized that what I was trained to do wasn't helping a large group of my patients. They were falling into a gaping hole in our healthcare system—they weren't critically ill (thankfully), but they weren't thriving either. Many women were being left and lost in a perpetual state of OK-ness. A state where they could sense they weren't actually OK, but no medical practitioner could tell them what was truly wrong. Why? Because they didn't neatly fit into a specific diagnostic test or medical label. They were caught in the mysterious abyss of the medical Bermuda Triangle, with no one to help or guide them. Many concluded that the problem was "in their head" or, even worse, that they were the problem.

This is how I discovered an ugly and daunting fact: our healthcare system is broken.

Because I've always thought of the symptoms of the body, no matter how big or small, as literal messages, I knew that chronic illness didn't just happen overnight. It was the result of dysfunction compounded over time. There was no way I was accepting "nothing wrong" as an answer. Plus, what was the alternative? Women discounting their symptoms as "just in their head" or believing their symptoms are "normal to feel as a woman"—I don't think so! This led them to stare down the barrel of discomfort and exacerbate distrust in their bodies, inevitably leading to medication or surgery as the only cure. Pardon my French but… FUCK that noise. Not on my watch.

So, this sparked another epic five-year journey to understanding what I was missing. I explored the medical field and completed a double masters in women's health medicine and reproductive medicine. I then further delved into functional health, studying functional medicine before looking into energetics through understanding breath work facilitation and Neuro Emotional Technique.

What I've learned from my unique experience studying across a broad range of health fields is that the system is set up to feed us fast food: empty, quick fixes that never quite hit the spot.

So… it's time for a new movement, a totally new wave of healthcare, because we deserve and hunger for something more. We're no longer satisfied with fast food style healthcare. I'm on a mission to plug that gaping hole women get lost in. To elevate them from quiet desperation to empowerment. I don't believe that women need to choose between two or three treatment options that don't even seem appealing. It's not OK for women to feel that they are destined for something to "go wrong": painful or heavy periods, miscarriages, infertility, fatigue, PMS, uncontrollable emotional waves, hysterectomies, pain medication, morning sickness, burning the insides of their organs, surgeries, medications that promise more freedom at the expense of their body's wisdom. And God forbid you don't experience any of these things, right? You could never say anything because then, worst of all, you'd be ostracized by other women, resulting in a shared warped sense of what's healthy, confusing "normal" with common.

Here's what we all need to know: the healthcare system is defined by conditions, labels, and treatments, so its essential framework works well for end-stage chronic illness, acute illness, and severe accidents. But is that what you're seeking help for? Most practitioners across all modalities are trained to think within the industry framework, to categorize diagnoses and label diseases. So, if you don't fit into the box they're looking through, essentially, they will say: "There's nothing wrong with you." Cause, well… you're not yet dying.

As a result, you're left feeling lost, unheard, and caught in limbo. Your body is telling you (or screaming at you) its needs. But because your symptoms don't tick their neat little diagnostic boxes, you're left unattended, without proper advice and support. You're being given fast food "fixes" instead of real solutions that focus on what your body needs.

So, if you've been labeled with a diagnosis of endometriosis, depression, fatigue, hormonal imbalance, autoimmune disease, gallstones—what does it mean for you?

It means that your body doesn't have what it needs.

Remember, your body is having a healthy response to an abnormal environment.

Yes, it's that simple! We've been made to feel like finding answers is too complicated. Like our body is broken. Like we're the issue. Like it's not worth trying because you'll just be dismissed, or perhaps you're too scared of what they might find. Scared to be labeled annoying just for being a woman. Again, fuck that noise!

On top of that, you're being bombarded by a sea of information that convinces you that you are the problem, perpetuated through social media, friends, family, health practitioners, TV, movies, pop culture, podcasts, and the like. No wonder we're left feeling confused and doubting the wisdom inside our bodies.

So, I'm here to give your health the makeover it so desperately needs (cue *Queer Eye* montage). Because when we understand what our bodies are telling us, it becomes a simple and exciting new way of relating to our bodies. We make health decisions based on our bodies' needs, not on what society is telling us.

We don't need to believe that the solutions to our health are complicated. I'm not buying it. I'm here to pioneer a simple and exciting new way forward. To bridge worlds that seem like they aren't connected. You see, I don't believe in black-and-white thinking. I believe that vibrant color is where the magic happens.

Think healthcare that isn't scary or complex, but fun even. Think cutting-edge technology and the wisdom of your body, guided by passionate, trained practitioners who use energetic, functional, and medical lenses. Yes, we exist!

I am here to help you feel your magic.

To remember your magic

To live your magic.

To know that your body isn't the problem—it's the solution.

Chapter 1

THERE'S NOTHING WRONG WITH YOU...

~

Surprise!

JANE IS JUST FINE

Let me tell you a little story about Jane. When Jane wakes up in the morning, she notices that she's still tired. She thinks, *I know how to fix that*, and makes herself a cup of coffee. When she washes her hair in the shower, she notices how much hair comes off her head. She thinks, *I know how to fix that*, and adds hair-strengthening shampoo to her grocery list. When she dries herself off, she notices how dry and scaly her skin is.

She thinks, *I know how to fix that*, and rubs moisturizer all over her body. When she sits on the toilet and her morning poo isn't coming, she thinks, *I know how to fix that*, and adds stool softener to her grocery list. After she's finished her breakfast and is on her way to work, she notices a wave of anxiety begin. She thinks, *I know how to fix that*, and remembers to take her antianxiety medication. When she notices white spots on her fingernails, she thinks, *I know how to fix that*, and paints her favorite red nail polish over the top. When her armpits keep sweating even though it's the middle of winter, she thinks, *I know how to fix that*, and sprays a thick coat of antiperspirant deodorant into her armpits. When she gets surprised by her irregular and quite heavy period, she thinks, *I know how to fix that*, and speaks to her doctor, who investigates and puts her on the pill.

Jane goes on living and feeling like she's thriving the best she can, keeping her body sticky taped together with a mixture of typical lifestyle fixes.

Years go by, and people comment on how lovely her nails are and how amazing her moisturizer must be. But when she forgets to renew her script, paint her nails, buy the shampoo, or take her medication, Jane notices she doesn't feel, or look, as good as she once did.

She's tired, losing hair, and her skin is dry and wrinkly. She's anxious and has started to develop skin rashes. Her periods have become even heavier, so much so she's beginning to bleed during the pill. Her body shape has changed, and, no matter how she adjusts her food or exercise, she can't seem to shift it. She speaks to her friends, and they verbalize similar difficulties or make light comments on how lucky she is that at least she doesn't also have a mustache. She speaks to her doctor, who does a round of tests, only to say there is nothing wrong with her. If she's "lucky," she'll be told she's anxious or depressed. Or that she's over exaggerating because her problems "aren't that bad" because "a lot of women feel like this." Jane is left to wait for her symptoms to get worse so she can go on medication or have surgery to solve her issues.

Jane's reality is the reality for millions of women worldwide every day. Millions of women are lost in the space between. Women who aren't dying but don't feel alive either.

~~~

Like Jane, many of us start off feeling and noticing small symptoms that the advertising industry has convinced us to be self-conscious about. Things like stretch marks, cellulite, acne, double chins, puffy ankles, bum pimples, tiredness, low sex drive. We see them as problems, markers that we're broken, that we need fixing, that there is something inherently wrong with us. That we should cover them up with a magic pill or tool that promises to leave us looking sexy, vibrant, and desired. It's no wonder we find it hard to feel worthy and safe in our bodies when we're constantly bombarded with messages that we need to be fixing some part of ourselves.

The amount of information we have access to now is unprecedented and can sometimes leave us second-guessing every little part of our lifestyles. What to eat for breakfast, what not to eat, how to exercise, or the next new biohack that promises us the world.

The rise and access to information is rampant, which in part is amazing because it helps to educate and raise awareness around certain issues that affect women specifically, things like endometriosis and PCOS for instance. But there comes a point when the awareness is so heightened that knowing someone who has a condition or experiencing a condition yourself is deemed "normal," instead of being seen as a message from the body that you (and also a lot of other people) need to change something you're doing so your body can be supported. This gap is exactly where women get lost in this perpetual state of "OK-ness."

~~~

The way I see it, women like Jane, who are lost in this space, currently have three options:

OPTION 1 – Accept that "there is nothing wrong" and ignore the signs their bodies are giving them. Wait for the symptoms to multiply or become more severe until finally they can be told there is something acutely wrong.

OPTION 2 – Push for the doctor to do something more or give them something for their symptoms.

OPTION 3 – Seek alternative help under their own guidance to hopefully find answers, and potentially get overwhelmed and not address the underlying cause, spending large sums of time and money trying to find what the fuck their bodies are trying to tell them.

Jane is all of us to some degree. We take the messages from our bodies for granted. We see them as a normal part of life. Of course, I'm tired in the morning—morning people are weirdos. Of course, I have stretch marks—everyone in my family does. Of course, I get a little PMS—that's normal for every woman. Then the symptoms can get a little louder and start to affect how our bodies function. We can get period pain that makes us bedridden for days, PMS that seriously affects our relationships and IBS that means we need to plan when and what we're eating, around access to a toilet.

We're looking through the lens of, *How can I make this go away or change my life to cope around my new normal?* We are holding our bodies together by tricking ourselves that it's all good, or that we can't do anything about it in the first place.

What if Jane viewed these small things that happen throughout the day as subtle messages from her body telling her what it needs?

What if Jane knew that waking up tired was a sign that one or several of her Female Fundamentals needed help? (more on this in Chapter 4).

Or her hair loss was a sign that her stress levels were impacting her sex hormone balance? Or the white spots on her fingernails were a sign her liver wasn't clearing copper sufficiently from her body, leading to higher estrogen levels, contributing to her heavy, painful periods? What if instead of hating these symptoms, she learned to love them? What if she understood that her amazing body was giving her the right signals to indicate what she needed to change in her life?

And, in fact, her symptoms were gifts?

Now I know what you're thinking. *Well, what the fuck? Am I just doing everything wrong? How am I meant to know what to do then? It seems like I can't do anything right. Is this doctor lady going to tell me I must move to a nudist colony in the hinterland of Byron Bay, where we all relish in our organic gardens and lady gardens, stinking like BO all day?*

No, I'm not going to tell you to do that. But by all means go and frolic in your birthday suit with *Pocketful of Sunshine* by Natasha Bedingfield playing in the background if that's what you want to do.

As you continue to read this book, you'll uncover a simple and fun way you can connect to your body, understand what it's telling you, and give it what it needs.

If you're looking for something that can slip into your lifestyle a little more seamlessly, you'll find a breakdown of common conditions and symptoms and what you can do about them in Chapter 3: "What's My Body Trying to Tell Me?"

Maybe these things you don't like about yourself or your body are exactly how your body is showing you that it loves you. Maybe your body is doing its best to adapt to the environment it's in. Maybe, as physician and author Gabor Maté says: "Disease is a normal response to an abnormal environment."[1] (You get that when I say maybe, I mean definitely, right?).

REAL MIRACLES HAPPEN EVERY DAY

The number one rule of the human body is balance. Balance between your external environment and your internal body environment is literally how we survive. So, every single millisecond, your body is making slight tweaks to your systems so it can adapt and survive. The fact that you're reading this right now means it's doing its job perfectly. Something as simple as sweating to cool you down when it's hot outside, or shivering to move your muscles and speed up your metabolism when you've stepped into a cool room, are examples of this process.

We can get so caught up in the next iPhone update, AI technology, or magical drugs promising to give us only positive thoughts or lose half our body weight without changing our lifestyles, that we forget that *we* are literally magic! And the very symptoms we don't like about ourselves are happening for a reason.

It's not that our bodies are working against us.
It's that they're always working for us.

You, right now—do you understand how miraculous it is that you're reading this? Trillions of automatic reactions are happening just to keep you alive. It's miraculous that your body knows when to wake up, and how to keep you alive and in a semiconscious state when you're asleep. It knows when to release your hormones and how to digest different foods. It remembers to breathe, make your heart beat, sweat, and keep your body temperature at a cool 36.5 degrees Celsius (or 97.7 degrees Fahrenheit). Don't even get me started on the odds of you being alive right now at this exact moment in time. And we think AI and the newest iPhone update are miracles. Please!

Let's look at this from a different perspective...

While you're sitting here reading or listening to this book, the fact that you can do this means, at the very least, that your eyes or your ears are working. Your brain is sending neural impulses connecting all of your senses and focusing your attention to then pair the words and information with the interconnected web of your own memory, formulating your perception of the content. Then a part of your brain called the frontal lobe performs its own judgment and perception of the content based on the information you believe to be true.

Each individual cell needs to have exactly what it needs to communicate with the cells around it, until these impulses form a pattern to create an action, habit, thought, or belief.

So, What Else is Happening Right Now?

Your heart is contracting and relaxing so blood can get to the areas it needs to for you to survive. Your postural muscles are contracting to keep you upright. Your gastrointestinal system is taking in the internal and external information to know how much stomach acid to produce—it effortlessly produces around 1.5 liters per day.

Your body is gauging the temperature outside and shifting things like your pulse rate, blood pressure, and stress hormones to know how much to sweat to keep your body temperature level. Your body temperature might have spiked slightly because you ovulated, or it might have increased a little so your body can burn off a current infection. (If that's the case, put the book down and grab some damn rest... We're not going anywhere. We'll be here when you feel better). Your brain is telling your thyroid, among other things, to speed up or slow down to make sure your cells are utilizing your available energy and using it wisely. Your pancreas is finding a fine balance between having enough sugar in your blood to maintain your energy but not so much that it's damaging to the rest of your body.

Your brain is telling your body to breathe. It's speeding up or slowing down depending on how much oxygen you have internally and the perceived demands in your external environment. Have you ever found yourself taking big, deep, slow breaths when you're hot? Yes, this is your body cooling you down and shifting your metabolism.

Oh, and by the way, all of these interactions are constantly interlinked with each other, sending messages back and forth so they know exactly how the other one is doing, if they need to make alterations to keep everything balanced and, importantly, your body alive. But this is just the tip of the iceberg.

What Has Happened Within the Last Day?

Well, you probably used your bowels without shitting yourself (hopefully). In fact, you might be on a plane at the moment thinking about how you need to do a poo and not wanting it to stink out the whole plane, so you're trying to hold it (girl, never hold it).

You might have had a tough conversation with someone, got the dream opportunity you've been working towards for months, hugged someone you love, lost someone you love… got stuck in traffic, felt like you were running out of time, felt like you were having the time of your life, wanted time to hurry up. You might have seen someone take their first steps, or their last, or you've had a birthday. (Happy birthday, by the way, you look amazing. If someone gave you this book as a gift, they have great taste). Maybe you went to work the same as you always do and wondered, *What the fuck am I going to cook for dinner tonight?* Or went to work and knew what you were having for dinner because you're a meal prep type of gal. Or went out and not worried about it because someone else does that for you. You might have run a marathon, or done a TV marathon. You might have heard someone talk about how they watched someone run a marathon, and now they're going to run one too.

Every single day is made up of these split-second moments, and these moments make up your life. There's one person who is always there for those moments, and that's you and your body. Your body is a constant. It's literally cheering you on every single moment until your dying breath. Because that's what it does.

That's what it has always done. Every time your heart beats, every time you take a breath, every time you release a hormone, have a menstrual cycle, and, yes, even when you do a poo, it's your body telling you that it's cheering you on, that it's here supporting you by keeping you alive.

The average lifespan of an Australian woman is 85 years.[2] That's 29,565 days. In that time...

- Her heart will beat 3.1 billion times (100,000 times per day).[3]
- She will take 620 million breaths (20,000 breaths per day).[4]
- She will secrete 46,537 liters of stomach acid (1.5 liters per day).[5]
- She will have on average 186 million thoughts (6,000 per day).[6]
- She will average around 450 menstrual cycles in her lifetime (providing she's not on contraceptives or has had surgeries that stop or mimic periods).[7]

Across every single moment, every single heartbeat, every single breath, your body has been cheering you on, doing everything it was designed to do to keep you alive, without you having to consciously think about it.

Please know that your body isn't broken. Quite the opposite. It's doing exactly what it was designed to do.

THE BUSINESS OF YOUR BODY

Think of your body like running a business, and the business has the best, most devoted employees ever. Your organs, tissues, and cells are the most highly trained and skilled personnel you could possibly ask for. They show up on time, always know what to do when, what to say, and how to fix issues before they even arise. They remember everyone's birthdays and favorite coffee order. They see opportunities and are always looking for growth. Any business owner would be chomping at the bit to have these guys working for them.

They'll do their best in pretty much any environment you put them in. They're programmed to work towards the same vision. They're self-managed experts, and they play well with others, adapting to change like champions to keep the business of your body alive.

But, as any good business owner knows, employees are only half of the equation. A supportive environment makes even the best employees even better. The trouble comes when the working conditions are lacking resources and make it hard for them to do their job properly—Try being an expert advertiser, coder, or salesperson without Wi-Fi, a laptop, or a phone. When we try to micromanage, stop listening to our employees, and start giving them what other business owners said was good for theirs, typically our employees (cells) get a little antsy. This is when we start to get bodily symptoms. If the working conditions continue to get tougher, although our employees are still highly skilled and trained to get the job done, they need to start cutting corners, sacrificing nonessential things for the essential. Just like when your business's bottom line is running a little skinny for the month and you skip out on the monthly business lunch, our bodies can skip a menstrual cycle or two because they're not essential to immediate survival. When you haven't been listening to your employees or haven't paid them fairly for their work, they go on strike. They can no longer handle the working conditions you've put them in, so they get vocal. This can look like autoimmune disease, chronic fatigue, IBS, cancer, or diabetes.

Without the belief and the trust that our employees know what they're doing, we think it's their fault. We haven't understood how to listen to what they're trying to tell us, or what the ideal working environment is for them. We listen to all the outside noise without checking in with them, with what they need. Remember—there's nothing wrong with the workers; they're telling you there's something wrong in their environment.

So, imagine if you were the owner of this business, and business performance was life or death. Wouldn't you want to be across everything? Wouldn't you want to understand what made your employees tick? What they really needed to feel supported? How to listen to and understand them? How to give them everything they needed to get the job done?

That's exactly what we need to do with our bodies.

When we understand that our bodies are literally magic, we start to look at them differently. We can understand that whether we have "good" skin or "bad" skin, feel energized or not, experience period pain, fatigue, stubborn weight gain, hair loss, IBS, autoimmune disease, migraines, and the plethora of health symptoms, or we feel amazing, all of these are side effects of our cells and our bodies having or lacking what they need to function.

So, when you're experiencing symptoms, or trying to find answers, and the result is either:

- A doctor or practitioner telling you there's nothing wrong with you.
- Hating your body because you don't like how you feel and nothing you've tried has worked.

Know that it's *not* a sign that your cells (employees) are broken. It's that you've made the working conditions hard for them, resulting in side effects because the workers are struggling to be as effective as they love to be.

You see, in a nutshell—**Your body is reflecting back to you what's going on inside.**

Does that mean you can't use skin care, moisturizer, nail polish, painkillers, or different clothes to help you feel better? Of course not. It just means understanding and knowing that your body is constantly giving you feedback on how it's liking its internal and external environment. When we use things that cover up this feedback, we can be lulled into a false sense of security, and these small changes can start to get bigger and bigger, eventually progressing into much larger issues.

This can be where we can start to trick ourselves.

DECODING OUR BODIES' MESSAGES (SYMPTOMS)

One of my patients, Lucy, is now 28 and came off the oral contraceptive pill two years ago. She first went on it at the age of 14 because her periods were painful and heavy. From the age of 14–26, she had painless and regular periods. When she turned 26, she had broken up with her partner and had decided she wanted to come off the pill "to give her body a rest."

In the two years since she came off the pill, her periods had been painful, heavy, and, in her words, "horrendous." Was it the pill's fault? Well, taking synthetic hormones orally for a long period of time does create knock-on effects with our guts, nutrient absorption, hormones, and all other systems of the body.[8] However, was it the pill that caused these issues, or was she already experiencing these symptoms beforehand? Remembering back to the reasons she went on the pill in the first place—they were the *exact* symptoms she was experiencing when she came off it. So, what does this tell us? We can't claim that the pill was to blame for causing her symptoms now, but what we can see is that her natural cycle hadn't changed since before she started the pill. This is a common trend that I often see in patients.

I also see patients who go on the pill for painful, irregular, or heavy periods and when they come off it, their periods are regular and non-painful. Was it the pill that "fixed" them, or was it that, in the time they were on the pill, their lifestyles changed? They changed what they were giving their bodies and when they finally came off the pill, they could use their natural menstrual cycles as a true measure of how their hormonal cycles were functioning in their bodies.

We must realize that the symptoms we have convinced ourselves are markers of our unworthiness, our brokenness, or signs that we need to hide parts of ourselves and hold ourselves together with duct tape because we're inherently fragile, *are actually signs that our bodies love us*. Signs that our bodies are strong and adaptable. Signs that are communicating exactly what our bodies need.

So, there's a fine line between understanding "there is nothing actually wrong with you" and "there is something actually wrong."

It's critical to investigate what our symptoms are trying to tell us, instead of ignoring them.

It's almost like we need to come full circle:

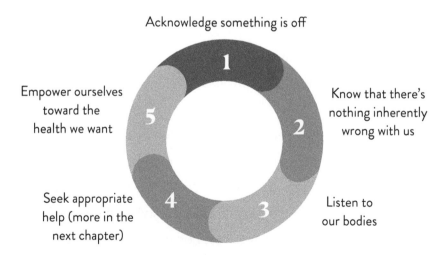

Are Your Symptoms Healthy, Normal, or Common?

Spoiler alert: common and normal are not actually the same thing. In fact, we have erroneously blended them together when they're poles apart. Let me explain…

Healthy—A sign that our bodies are loving us.

Normal—What we think is healthy because it's common but actually is a sign from our bodies that they need support.

Common—Things that are common that we know aren't healthy.

It's common to think that being a woman means we're going to hate our bodies for one reason or another. Either they don't look the way they're supposed to, or they don't do what they're supposed to. It's common, but not normal.

We consider it normal to suffer with gut issues, but it's not healthy. Depression has become so common it's normal, but is having 280 million people in the world diagnosed with it normal, or does it highlight a greater issue?[9]

Is it normal to think you might have fertility issues? Do we need to be aware that everyone has different fertility journeys? Yes. Do we need to be aware of what our bodies need to support a pregnancy? Yes. Is it normal to think that you'll struggle with fertility? No. It is common though.

Is it normal to dread menopause? It's unrealistic to think that we should care for our bodies the same way at 50 as we did at 20. It's common to dread menopause, but it's not normal.

Just because we don't know what we need to change, it doesn't mean we're doomed to feel like we're drowning in a sea of terrible symptoms.

~

Let's play a quick game to find out. Run through the following list of symptoms and tell me if they're healthy, normal, or common. Just go off your gut instinct.

- Acne
- PMS
- Anxiety
- Depression
- Mix of emotions
- Bloating
- Tired when you wake up
- Cancer
- Falling asleep as soon as you sit down
- 5-day bleed of your menstrual cycle
- 25-day menstrual cycle
- Stretch marks
- Diabetes
- Doing a poo every second day
- Floating poo
- Taking 5–15 minutes to fall asleep at night
- Brown blood at the start of your period

We'll be going more into these in the coming chapters. For now, it's cool to understand what our base mindset is.

Healthy	Normal	Common
Mix of emotions	PMS	Anxiety
5-day bleed of your menstrual cycle	Tired when you wake up	Depression
Taking 5–15 minutes to fall asleep at night	Brown blood at the start of your period	Cancer
25-day menstrual cycle	Bloating	Diabetes
	Stretch marks	Acne
	Doing a poo every second day	Falling asleep as soon as you sit down
	Floating poo	

What is *Your* Normal?

When we allow "common" and "normal" to infiltrate our thoughts on what's healthy, we come to know and develop our own concept of "normal." That's why so many of us have a different normal.

We live different lives; we're from different cultures and backgrounds; our parents, friends, and families all grew up with different traditions, different jobs, different incomes. What we do and who we surround ourselves with is different. This puts us in different circumstances, allowing our perceptions of normal to change.

For instance… one of my friends would play cards or read with her family after dinner. This was normal for her. I, on the other hand, would watch medical shows. She will whoop your butt in a game of cards and is an amazing writer, and I love understanding people's bodies.

One of my other friends would have bottles of soft drink at the table for dinner. This was their normal because it's what they commonly did. I didn't see it as healthy, although the teenage version of me did love a treat when I would visit.

One of my other friends has a family tradition where they do a family 10 km (6 mile) run on Christmas morning. For them, it's normal. For me and my family, we have chocolate for breakfast in our pajamas while unwrapping presents. For other families, Christmas isn't celebrated.

Our perception of what is normal
is altered by what is *common* for us.

The same is true for our health. Our perception of what is healthy is altered when we allow the common to create our "norm."

You might be thinking, *Why does this matter?* Because when we get these terms confused, we can miss messages from our bodies telling us that we need to change something. When these messages go unmet, they get loud.

I've met and cared for a lot of people who have experienced various forms of cancer in their lives either personally or with their loved ones. Earlier this year, I met a 23-year-old who had been diagnosed with breast cancer. As you can imagine, it turned her whole life upside down in an instant. Being told you have something that people equate to death is probably one of the most confronting things anyone will face, let alone a 23-year-old. But what she said and how she related to the news really stuck with me.

She decided that the cancer wasn't a sign that her body was weak, disease-ridden, or broken. She decided that it was a message from her body. It was a big wake-up call. It was her body's way of saying she needed to drastically change what she was doing, thinking, and being because it was literally killing her. Essentially, her body was having a healthy response to an abnormal environment.

So, what did she do?

She quit her job; she moved states; she changed how she was thinking, what she was eating, and connected with her friends, family, and her body. She let her body lead her to what she needed to do.

This girl, although amazing in her own right, isn't special. There are countless accounts of people who have been diagnosed with cancer and have gone into remission or survived "against all odds" because they used it not as a message that they were broken, but as a message (a shouting one) that they needed to change some things in their lives.

AUTOMATIC SYSTEMS OF THE BODY —THE ELEPHANT IN THE ROOM

Are you doing all the biohacking, meditation, breathwork, exercising, and diets because you're trying to fix a part of yourself that you hate? Or because you love how it nourishes your body?

The difference can look something like:

- *I just don't want to feel tired today* **versus** *I want to feel energized today.*
- *I must do my morning meditation because I hate that I'm anxious* **versus** *I'm doing my morning meditation because I love connecting to my body and having this time just for me.*
- *I'm going to the gym so I look fit and skinny* **versus** *I'm going to the gym because I love how strong my body feels when I work out.*
- *My body is defective* **versus** *My body is amazing and is giving me these symptoms to tell me how to support it.*

See the difference?

I used to be cynical about "the power of intention." I often thought, *Even if I set the intention for what I want, it doesn't mean I'll get it.*

But I soon realized there's a slight shift with intention that makes a big difference. It's all around focusing on what you do want, as opposed to focusing on what you don't want. Simple, right?

When we focus on what we want, our brains automatically wire to look for and find things that agree with that reality, that is, our intention. We see this all the time, and, in science, it's often referred to as confirmation bias. Basically, when we already have a belief, our brains only pay attention to the information that reinforces that belief.

The healthcare and advertising industries are set up to look for what isn't working—to "hunt" for symptoms—and when they find them, it's confirmation that there is something wrong with you, which is often confirmed by putting a label or diagnosis onto those symptoms. It's proof that you are broken, right?

Let's look at it another way…

Let's take, for instance, stubborn weight around your mid-section. You might go to the doctors and have a series of tests done, looking into your cholesterol, blood sugars, blood cells, and thyroid. All of which more than likely will come back "normal."

I see time and time again women who struggle with this issue, who practically starve themselves and work themselves into the ground at the gym to try and lose the weight, but it just won't shift. So, when nothing we do to "fix" ourselves works and the doctors have said, "There's nothing wrong with you," there aren't many other mental spaces to go to other than, *I must be broken.*

Unless…

We remember that our bodies always have clear and clean intentions, even if we're experiencing symptoms or diseases we don't like. Our bodies are always changing and adapting for a reason. So, when you experience a symptom or have been diagnosed with a condition, ask yourself, *Why does my body think this is the best thing to do?*

Weight gain around the abdomen provides protection for our vital organs. It often becomes stubborn when our stress levels have been high for a prolonged period of time and a whole hormonal cascade occurs, leading to abdominal fat to protect us and our vital organs.

Acne can be how our bodies tell us we have poor detoxification internally and that we need to detox through the skin. It can also signify that we need to support our own boundaries, because our skin is a physical boundary of our bodies. Your body doesn't *want* to leave you looking all scarred and pimply. It's telling you your Fundamentals are off (more on this in Chapter 4).

I find it useful to get still and calm and gently ask the part of your body, *What are you telling me?* The answer might surprise you.

And before you think, *My body is going to tell me I'm fat and ugly*, remember…your body is your biggest cheerleader. Cheerleaders are always supportive. Our bodies don't intend to do us harm. They have pure intentions. When we understand this, we can also alter our own intentions so we can work with our bodies, instead of against them.

⌒

This book isn't going to tell you that all you need to do is think there's nothing wrong with you, and all of your health and life problems will be miraculously solved. If that were the case, the title of the book would be *God Complexes—the New Health Trend*.

What I intend this book to do is help you cultivate a deep trust in yourself and in your body. Because, really, they are the same thing. I intend for you to connect to your inherent wisdom. You may have become disconnected because of traumas that made you disassociate from your body as a coping mechanism and trust others more than you trust yourself, or because you've been conditioned to listen to society and alter your actions to fit in. A society and system that often makes our bodies out to be the enemy when, really, they're the solution. We've made it common to believe that our bodies are stopping us from living our best lives rather than telling us how to live our best lives. We try to squish our bodies into our lifestyles with all of the biohacks under the sun instead of our lifestyles into our bodies.

So, even if you're doing "all the right things"—the breath-work, the dieting, the supplements, the saunas and cold plunges, listening to the podcasts with brand-new research—remember why you are doing it. Remember that the number one goal is to give your body what it needs (the Female Fundamentals™). When we do that, we work in alignment with the pure intentions of our bodies, and the symptoms we've been fighting begin to melt away.

Warning: The power of intention does not give you the skills to perform a backflip if you have not tried it before. Batteries not included. Terms and conditions apply.

The very belief that you must keep fixing yourself to get what you want could be the very thing stopping you from experiencing what you want.

Side note: In the beginning, this can be a big shift in percep-tion. Know that you can hold both the old feeling that you're broken with the new belief that your body is working for you at the same time. Kind of like when your child annoys you by throwing a tantrum in the middle of the supermarket aisle, yet you still love them deeply. You can make room for both.

Everything your body is doing,
it is doing it *for* you, *not* against you.
Your body doesn't do *anything* against you.
Your body doesn't do anything just for
the sake of inconveniencing you.

So, the next time you're told there's nothing wrong with you…

Ask yourself, *How is this benefiting me? What's my body trying to tell me?*

Chapter 2

THE HEALTH SPECTRUM

~

The space between black and white isn't gray;
it's color...that's the magic.

LET YOUR BODY BE YOUR GUIDE

Often, when we decide to visit a healthcare practitioner, the type of practitioner we select depends on what beliefs we grew up with. I've seen people who have never been to a medical practitioner before because they "don't trust them" but when they take antibiotics for their chronic infection, they get better. I've also cared for patients who have put up with chronic back pain and dysfunction for years and who couldn't believe they waited so long to get chiropractic care.

The beauty of modern-day life is that a lot of us have access to a range of medical, functional, and energetic practitioners. The key is to know what type of care you need, using your body, not your bias, as a guide.

Illness Happens Over Time

Recently, I started seeing a patient—let's call her Sammy. Sammy works in a hospital and is a 36-year-old woman with a plethora of symptoms. She was suffering from postural orthostatic tachycardia syndrome (POTS), which is when your heart rate goes into a different rhythm and beats incredibly fast when you sit or stand up, causing you to feel dizzy, exhausted, and sometimes faint. For her, it only occurred when she was pregnant, requiring her to take heart-rate-lowering medication throughout her pregnancies.

She was also diagnosed with endometriosis. Her hair was thinning, and she was exhausted, in chronic pain, and couldn't use her bowels unless she gave herself a coffee enema every morning. She was constantly battling with her internal mind and her body, wanting to play with her young children and live a great life but riddled with guilt because her body often felt like it was holding her back. She's strong though. She has the kind of personality you would want by your side in the good times and the bad times. That strong friend who you often forget to check in on.

She is also incredibly smart and knew that how she was feeling wasn't normal. She had sought out further investigations to make sure nothing "really bad" was going on, visiting amazing cardiologists, endocrinologists, and gynecologists. What did they all say?

- **Cardiologist (heart specialist):** "It's not a heart issue because it comes out when your hormones shift. See an endocrinologist."
- **Endocrinologist (hormone specialist):** "It's not a hormone thing, your thyroid is fine. See your cardiologist for your heart or gynecologist for the endo."
- **Gynecologist (women's reproductive organ and hormone specialist):** "POTS is a cardiologist thing. If your endo keeps giving you pain or you keep losing too much menstrual blood, we can cut out your uterus, because you're done having kids."

Are any of these doctors "bad" doctors? No, not at all.

In fact, we funnily realized that her cardiologist was the very professor that operated on my heart all those years ago. So, in this case, I can personally say he is very good at what he does and there wouldn't be many other people I would want poking around my heart.

So, where did that leave Sammy? She hadn't been able to get any answers, even when she saw "the best of the best." She was given treatment options that treated her symptoms but didn't explain to her "why" she was experiencing what she was experiencing.

So, she, like so many other women, as I see it, only had three options:

OPTION 1 – Resign herself to the fact that this was her "new normal" and she would eventually end up waiting for the symptoms to get bad enough for some kind of surgery or medication change.

OPTION 2 – Carry out the current treatment options even though there weren't any she liked—but hey, something's better than nothing, right?

OPTION 3 – Listen to her body and keep looking for someone or something to help make sense of what her body was trying to say and make changes to support her whole body.

～

Sammy was a lot like most of the patients I see. Often feeling alone and losing hope that life could be any different. Losing trust in their bodies and making themselves out to be the issue. Resigning themselves to the fact that this must be their new reality.

But there is one thing that sticks out with people like Sammy: they still have a connection to that little voice inside them saying, *There is something you're missing.* They still have enough hope and trust in their bodies to keep looking for someone or something to help them find answers.

They're the ones who took option three. The ones who let the voice of their bodies shine through a little louder than the voice of doubt. Instead of the voice of, *There is no other option,* the voice of, *You're just broken*, it's the voice of, *I'm trying to tell you something,* the voice of, *I've got you, keep paying attention*, the voice of, *You're not broken, this is happening for a reason.*

When you have the belief that your body isn't the problem— it's the solution—you take option three every time.

When I sat down with Sammy and reviewed her whole health history and timeline, she mentioned that the fast heart rate and dizziness (POTS) was triggered in pregnancy. At the end of our first consultation, I could see the hope start to creep back into her face. I could see that she was no longer resigning herself to the fact that she was broken or that she couldn't find the answers she needed.

I said to her, "You don't grow endometrial tissue out of nowhere. You don't develop POTS out of nowhere. What if we were to view all these symptoms as a way your body is working *for* you? A way that it is coping and keeping you alive given your changing circumstances? *A healthy response to an abnormal environment?*"

When we traced it back, she noted that, in high school, she always had a much faster heart rate than her classmates. So, even though her heart issues were exacerbated by the changes in hormones and proteins in her pregnancy, the heart rate issues could have been there earlier.

When I asked her about what had happened or was happening in her life around that time in her younger years, she shared that a traumatic, life-threatening event had occurred to her, and her father still had nightmares about it. This was followed by the sudden death of a relative and ongoing threats to her safety in the year proceeding. It made sense that her body was feeling how it was feeling.

But Should You *Always* Take Option Three?

What if you need medical care and treatment? To understand the answer, we need to understand the evolution of healthcare. If we think back to the 1920s, the leading cause of death was largely due to infections—things like typhoid fever, malaria, measles, dysentery, and scarlet fever. In the 1920s, water sanitation started to change in the United States, and the number of deaths due to these waterborne infections dropped dramatically. It was in 1928 that penicillin, the first mainstream antibiotic, was discovered, with mass production beginning in the mid 1940s.[10] This, in combination with better sanitation, drastically reduced the number of deaths caused by infectious diseases, which was the leading cause of death at the time.

Fast-forward to modern health statistics. The top five leading causes of death in Australia are coronary artery disease, stroke, chronic obstructive pulmonary disease, lung cancer, and dementia.[11] What do all of these conditions have in common? You can't catch them or give them to someone else. If I have a stroke and you come near me, it doesn't mean you run the risk of having a stroke too. It doesn't take a rocket scientist to recognize that these main causes of death and disability need a completely different framework of thinking if we want to address the underlying cause. It's a whole different ball game. Like trying to play basketball with tennis rules. It just doesn't make sense to treat chronic illnesses like we do acute ones.

We've made our roads safer, our hygiene better, but we haven't changed the way we think about our health.

We're using an acute illness mindset to try and address chronic illnesses. If we can't see it or test for it, like we can with an infection or a broken arm, then it mustn't exist. So, we allow the dysfunction to continue to creep in and creep in; we alter what we think of as "healthy" by society's standards, and then, all of a sudden, seemingly out of nowhere, we're diagnosed with a chronic illness. No, no, no. This works for acute illness because they're usually quick and require short treatment. If you have a broken arm, you have surgery or put your arm in a cast, wait six weeks, and you're back to functioning. If you get bacterial meningitis, you receive antibiotics (early enough); the infection is cleared, and you go on living your life.

If you get type 2 diabetes, you start taking medication, but it doesn't clear up. The dysfunction is still there, so you then keep taking medication for the rest of your life… If you have irregular cycles, you take medication to make them regular. When you stop the medication, the irregular cycles can return, for the rest of your life…

This isn't how it works.
Chronic illness, by definition, happens over time.

We're conditioned to miss the whispers. For instance, did you know that more than half of women with PCOS will develop diabetes by the time they're 40.[12] How do we treat PCOS at the moment? It's based around caring for your different symptoms. The pill is used to artificially regulate your periods and blocks hormones contributing to acne. Laser hair removal is used for excess hair growth, and it's recommended to lose weight either with medication or lifestyle change. We're in the mindset of shutting down the symptom and getting rid of the "damn" things. Irregular periods are annoying. Chin hair and nipple hair are annoying and gross—get rid of them.

Except irregular periods and chin hairs aren't some external bacteria coming to get you. The "get rid of them" mentality is great with acute illness because it is an external pathogen infiltrating our system. But when we use the same get rid of them mentality to shut down the messages and symptoms from within the body, we end up blocking the solution to our problems because we see it as the enemy. Not only that, but we're unconsciously conditioning ourselves to view our bodies as the enemy. Your body is *never* the enemy, especially when it comes to chronic illness.

We're missing the warning signs of chronic illness because we've normalized the warning signs.

You want to know how to address chronic illness? Pay attention to what your body is telling you. Know that it's *normal* to feel healthy. It's *normal* to listen to your body and make decisions based on what your body needs. It's *normal* to trust what your body is telling you. It's *normal* to be proactive, give your body what it needs, and then let it do its thing.

YOU'VE GOT ZEBRAS IN YOUR KITCHEN

The way the healthcare system is set up now is all about *what* is going on with you. And by *what*, I mean, can we give you a name, a label, for what you're feeling or experiencing?

When a name, label, or diagnosis can be given to what you're experiencing, there can be a code attached to your name. This code enables funding to be given from the medical system. It also enables rebates on different drugs and services, and it makes it easier to communicate across practitioners. Having a label or someone actually tell you what is happening is brilliant. In the beginning. It's validating, it makes you feel like you're not going crazy.

It's kind of like this. Imagine you're sitting in your kitchen, and there's a zebra eating food from your fridge. You call the zoo wrangler and say, "Come and get this zebra."

They arrive and, after having a look around, say, "I don't know what you're talking about. There's no zebra here. It's in your head, just go buy some more food."

You call a different wrangler, and they say the same thing. So, you start to become a little disheartened and go and buy some more food.

The zebra comes back, and this time brings more of its friends. You've now got an elephant and giraffe helping themselves to your pantry. You call the wrangler, and finally they see that you have an issue. "Oh, you have a big problem. We need to get rid of these animals and take them back to the zoo."

In the beginning, it's great. You get rid of them. But did anyone stop to look at how they got into your house in the first place? Or were they so busy fixing the problem of the zoo in your kitchen that they didn't realize you had turned your backyard into a zoo?

So, when we're finally told, "Yes, there is something wrong with you," it can be nice in the beginning. It's validating. It makes us feel like we're not going crazy, and it's not just in our head. But how backwards is that? To be happy that someone says there's something inherently broken with you. We feel relieved that there's a reason for what we're experiencing that's external to us. This thought process is amazing when we have an acute illness, infection, or accident because often the cause is largely external. However, when we're struggling with conditions like autoimmune disease, endometriosis, cancer, or diabetes, the cause isn't formed externally; it's formed internally as a response to chronic adaptive patterns from the body. A healthy response to an abnormal environment.

～

So, how do we get to the point where we can acknowledge that what's happening is a sign that our bodies are in fact not broken? They've simply been responding how they've needed to for survival. This doesn't mean we're locked into this forever. It's lovely to be validated, but it doesn't really solve the underlying issue.

Have you ever found yourself saying…

- "I'm never going back to the doctor. I don't trust them."
- "'I can't believe Suzie down the road won't go and get antibiotics for that terrible cough she's had for months."
- "My sister is into all this woo-woo crap now."

As a practitioner I've heard people on all sides of the fence. You hate medicine and think it's the devil, and you don't trust doctors "as far as you can kick them," or you think that medicine is the "only way."

Long-term health exists on a spectrum. It's constantly shifting and changing. Where we sit on the spectrum depends on a couple of things. The internal and external environments we put our bodies in, and how long they've been there.

Our bodies are super adaptable. Even when you think someone is the most rigid person in the whole world, their body is still adapting. It has to in order to survive. When we stop adapting is when we die. Our symptoms are feedback from our bodies highlighting how they've decided to adapt and how well that adaptation is going.

WHAT IF THERE'S NO HELP OR ANSWERS?

So, what do you do if you've reached out for help and haven't received answers for why you feel how you feel? What do you do next?

First of all, it's annoying, right? As a practitioner, I understand this from the other side too—the frustration of seeing a patient suffering or experiencing a bunch of symptoms and referring them for testing and investigation only to seemingly find nothing on their tests. We know you want answers, and we want to give them to you. Unfortunately, because of how the system is set up, if there are symptoms but no hard evidence on tests, we're told there's nothing wrong; it's in our heads. Or we're basically told to wait until we're bad enough to seek help. *What the fuck?!*

The most heartbreaking thing I see and experience with patients is when they're told there's nothing wrong with them or they're given options for treatment that all seem "terrible" and they don't want to choose any of them.

This happened enough in just my first couple of years of working that I needed to find answers. I could no longer bear seeing the look of hopelessness and despair on my patients' faces. So, over several years, I studied across medical, functional, and energetic fields to encapsulate what I call the health spectrum. I developed an understanding that patients need access to all forms of guidance and tools, depending on where they sit on the spectrum at the time. When one modality says, "There's nothing wrong," it just means we need to use a different approach.

On the Chiropractic side, we're taught to do something called "differential diagnosis", which is where we understand when we can help someone and when we need to refer them to another health practitioner. Typically, this means medical attention. After several years of referring female patients to their medical practitioners and seeing them return feeling deflated, I thought maybe the doctors didn't know what they were talking about. I fell into the trap of thinking it was the person, not the system. What I discovered after studying my double master's in women's health and reproductive medicine was that "the space between" wasn't a thing. You either had something, or you didn't. A great model when we're looking at acute illness, not so great when assessing chronic illness.

So, if you're a woman who feels "lost in the space between," like you have no idea what your body is telling you, and your doctors don't seem to have any answers for you—keep reading.

~~~

It's like if you tried to use a telescope instead of a microscope to look inside a cell. You'd think that nothing as small as a cell existed. Similarly, you wouldn't think space existed if you were trying to use a microscope to see it. It's the same when we use the wrong instruments, tests, and approaches for what we want to view. If you want to look for disease that's already happening, use medical testing. If you want to look at dysfunction and the *why*, you need functional testing. If you want to understand the subconscious patterns in your life that are creating your reality and physical manifestation of health, use an energetic approach. Both the telescope and microscope are important, depending on the context.

Context is how women keep falling through the cracks. We get told things like:

- "Of course you're tired and depressed. You have young kids you're running around after."
- "You just need to look at the big picture, and you'll be less anxious."
- "You're just lazy. That's why you're tired."

(Yes, these are real life examples from patients).

I can tell you that all the women I see aren't making it up. They want the best for their bodies. They just don't know where the fuck to start.

If that's you, start by finding a practitioner who's the perfect match. In your search for answers, it's important to understand what type of help you need and when.

YOUR RELATIONSHIP TO HEALTH

Hands up if you've been personally victimized by the healthcare system? Regina George? If you don't know this reference, then for goodness' sake please do yourself a favor and watch *Mean Girls*. It's a classic 2004 movie.

For those who (God-forbid) haven't seen this chick flick, then let me give you a quick recap and explain what the names

Regina George and Aaron Samuels have to do with your health. You see, Regina and Aaron were the two most popular teens in school, and it made sense that these two gorgeous, baby-faced teens should get together and be the all-American couple. BUT once you look deeper—well, as deep as *Mean Girls* can go—you can see that their pairing is way off. They don't have much in common, but everyone thinks they make the ultimate power couple.

When they finally take a sober look and stop and ask themselves why they're together in the first place, it's pretty obvious they have nothing in common and really should break up. It was fun while it lasted, but it would be best for them to go their different ways.

You and the healthcare system may have the same type of relationship as Regina and Aaron. Deep, I know. On the surface, you and the current healthcare system may look like the perfect match. But scratch a little deeper, and you may not be as compatible as the posters on the wall at the doctor's office like to suggest.

It's the same when we have chronic non-life-threatening conditions or symptoms that we deem as "normal," things like, endometriosis, PCOS, acne, painful periods, PMS, poor sleep, brain fog, stretch marks, white spots on our fingernails, recurrent injuries, and chronic headaches. Some of these conditions like to hang out with Regina, but the relationship goes nowhere fast. When we look at why they're happening, we can pair them with someone functional. In this case, Cady Heron, aka Lindsay

Lohan. Then they can be themselves and have a relationship that works best for them.

Now, was it that any of the characters didn't deserve love or that one person was better than the other? Not at all. In fact, quite the opposite. When all of the characters stopped trying to be someone else, stopped trying to make a relationship work that clearly wasn't the right pairing, they got exactly what they needed. They all had a better suited match. Even Regina George.

The key was that they needed to know who their better match was.

It's the same with healthcare. I've seen and heard countless patients have different perspectives on the same circumstance. Look at what happened to the world during COVID. It divided people. It made it feel like people were pressured to choose between one or the other. There was no room for both. No room for nuance. The body is FULL of nuance. That's literally it's job. It's like saying everyone needs to be dating Aaron Samuels. What if your dad's name is Aaron and you can't bear the thought of kissing someone with the same name? See, nuance.

The issue isn't the healthcare methods and training. It most likely isn't that your doctor is crap and doesn't know what they're talking about. Or that energy workers are full of shit and playing mind games on you. Or that your chiropractor just took your money and didn't fix your migraines. Most of the time, the practitioners are highly skilled at what they do. Granted, it's a service industry, so at times it will be hit-and-miss. Just like getting a great haircut from one hairdresser and coming out looking like Donald Trump another time (this actually happened to me as a child because of chronic head lice... a story for another day).

They're all amazing and needed. The issue is that we've mismatched them. Or we only see the popular girl or guy as worthy of love and attention, so if you're not a match for her, you don't need any support, right? It must be in your head, right? Being forced to see the world in black and white is a great way to feel pressured and fearful. When it comes to healthcare and a lot of other parts of life, know that you can take the bits you like, you can change your mind, you can sit with what feels right to you, you color within your own lines. When we do this, we're leading from the wisdom of the body.

~~~

If you're not loving your health or your life at the moment, or you feel like you've been victimized by the healthcare industry, it's a sign that you need to play matchmaker with yourself.

Maybe the things happening in your life aren't actually making you feel how you thought you'd feel. Maybe you've always wanted to feel fit and strong, and, after eight weeks of running, you're still hating your life, and all you have to show for your effort is injury after injury. Maybe you're back and forth to the doctor's office with recurrent respiratory issues, and, no matter the investigations and medication, nothing seems to be helping. Maybe you're constipated, backed up to the hilt, and the only thing that works for you is laxatives every day. You know that when you stop, the constipation will start again. Maybe you've taken all the supplements, altered your morning routine to include breathwork, meditation and protein, but you're still exhausted because you can't bring yourself to ask for help. You're doing the work of an entire household by yourself, seeing it as weak or feeling guilty when you need help.

This may seem a little bit pedantic, but, just like it's important to be on the same page as the person you're dating, it's important to find the type of healthcare that suits you. To do that, you need to understand where you're sitting on the health spectrum. How do you know if there really is nothing sinister going on? How do you know if you have the right practitioner matched to your symptoms?

Just like you wouldn't see your dentist for your bowel cancer or your nutritionist when you're having a heart attack, should we not question why we would use current medical thinking of drugs and surgery to address the root cause of something that's chronic, underlying, and non-life-threatening? Endometriosis, IBS, acne, hypothyroidism, painful period, anxiety—these conditions start out as functional issues and, only after long-standing dysfunction, progress to a point of needing medication.

To find the type of care you need, I like to split the healthcare system into three sections: **energetic**, **functional**, and **medical**.

This is when we need to play matchmaker. When we have a condition that needs functional support and we're just using energetics, it's like partnering Aaron Samuels with Gretchen Wieners. It's OK, but there's something missing.

Our bodies talk to us on the spectrum of energetic, functional, and medical. It depends on how severe and how long-standing the message is. The same message can keep appearing until it gets louder and louder and louder. If we don't address it, or tend to it, it doesn't go away; it just manifests itself in other ways.

MAEVE, MINERALS, AND MEDICINE

One of my patients, let's call her Maeve, was a 21-year-old who experienced irregular periods, ranging anywhere from 45–65 days between bleeds. She also had cystic acne, and her blood test results indicated a significant thyroid issue. Her medical doctor suggested she start on medication straight away and that she would need to be on it for the rest of her life. After reviewing her blood and test results, I did agree that, given her symptoms, her thyroid was under significant distress. What we didn't know was why, and what we knew was a lifetime of medication didn't sound like a solution at all.

So, we went looking into her functional health. In her case, we used a hair tissue mineral analysis, which is a great test for looking at the function of your body and assessing all four of your Female Fundamentals (which we dive into in Chapter 4). We found that three of her four Female Fundamentals needed direct assistance. Nutrient wise, she had very low levels of potassium, which was making it difficult for her thyroid and cells to generate energy, alongside her arsenic levels being well above normal limits, blocking her thyroid from being able to produce active thyroid hormone. Although she had a great diet, which supported her blood sugar Fundamental, her ability to absorb nutrients and excrete toxins was being affected. We needed to support her nervous system to boost her production of stomach acid and absorption while digesting the nutrients from the supplements her body needed. These steps aimed to reduce her overall inflammation. Lastly, we made changes to her exercise, eating times, and sunlight routine to actively support her metabolism.

After three months of lifestyle changes in line with the Female Fundamentals and specific supplement changes, her medical tests showed that her thyroid levels had returned to normal, and her functional hair test illustrated marked improvements in her thyroid, adrenals, arsenic levels, and liver function. Her cycles and basal body temperature for measuring ovulation became more frequent, and her overall skin and energy levels drastically improved. Going to show, it's important to look at your symptoms and test results as messages from the body. It's not that you're broken, but quite the opposite—your body is telling you how and where it needs support.

I recently received an email from Maeve letting me know that she and her partner were over the moon because they just found out she was pregnant!

DOES THAT MEAN YOU ALWAYS NEED TO AVOID MEDICINE?

I had a woman reach out to me to see if I could help her. She had been heavily bleeding menstrually for six weeks straight. She'd been to her doctor, and the drugs she had originally been given had stopped working after one week. Did that mean that applying a functional or energetic approach was what she needed? Maybe so, but not right now. For her, no amount of functional or energetic work could outweigh the blood loss she was experiencing at the time. Once the bleeding had stopped and she had been investigated for life-threatening causes of the bleeding and her body had regained a basic level of function, then we could start to look into functional and energetic causes. But it's dangerous and counterproductive to use that type of care in this circumstance. Remember, to give your body what it needs, you should match your symptoms with the *correct type* of healthcare.

ENERGETIC, FUNCTIONAL, AND MEDICAL

Energetic—*What we can't see creates what we can see.*

What is Energetics?

Energetics can be an abstract concept to wrap our head around, because we can't see it. You might be someone who is highly attuned or someone who is as deaf as your grandad when it comes to tuning into the subtleties of your body.

Much like we can't see Wi-Fi or the radio waves from our phones when we make a phone call, our energetics are unseen, but they are creating the frequency that our cells vibrate on, which alters how we perceive our reality.[13]

Common signs you may notice energetically

- You feel stuck.
- You feel bliss.
- You're replaying patterns.
- You feel magnetized to do something but can't consciously explain why.
- You don't know where you're going.
- You don't feel like you have control over your life.
- It's difficult to verbalize how you feel.
- You notice that your voice cracks or goes when you're not sure about something.
- You feel "out of your body"—always in a rush, speaking fast, walking fast.
- Mental chatter runs wild.
- You feel your body want to shake or move throughout the day.
- You often have feelings you can't cognitively explain.

When is the best time to use it?

All the time. No matter if you have a chronic illness or acute illness, focusing on your energetics is beneficial every day. However, when we start to experience physical symptoms, we need to start using the other approaches alongside our energetics.

Tools and guidance for this approach

Practitioners trained in connecting you to your body and releasing unconscious patterns (this is a brief, profound list, although there are many other forms):

- Kinesiology
- Somatic healing
- Neuro-emotional technique
- German New Medicine
- Spinal energetics

Tools you can use

- Daily embodiment practice and making decisions based on intuition
- The power of intention
- Energetic boundaries
- Paying attention to the stories we tell ourselves

Hint: If you can explain your intuition… it's not your intuition.

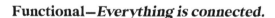

Functional—*Everything is connected.*

What is Functional?

Functional is everything your body requires for its physiology to work. It's understanding that all parts of the body are connected and influence each other.

Common signs and symptoms
(this list is comprehensive but not complete)

- Frequently feeling tired
- Rashes or acne
- Bloating
- PMS
- Painful periods
- Anxiety
- Depression
- Excessive sweating
- Being told to not worry about doing anything about your symptoms until you can't put up with them anymore
- Menopausal hot flashes
- Difficulty losing weight

When is the best time to use it?

- You have symptoms that can't be tested using "typical testing." Think about all the conditions that can't be shown on scans or blood tests. Think acne, anxiety, depression, hair loss, IBS, and so on.
- You have a chronic illness or symptoms and want to understand why.
- You have been told there is "nothing wrong" on your medical tests but still feel like there's something wrong.

Tools and guidance for this approach

- Use your 4 Female Fundamentals (we're diving deep into this in Chapter 4).
- Understand what your physical body symptoms are telling you (Chapter 3).
- Find a Practitioner who can help guide you.

~~~

Medical—*It doesn't exist unless we can see it or test for it.*

What is Medical?

You can think of medical as the traditional, westernized medical system, where you use a general practitioner or physician as the main port of call and for referrals for further testing or medication.

Common traits of medical

- It doesn't exist unless you can see it.
- Seeking to identify a condition physically, on a test or diagnostic criterion.
- The business of labeling.
- Disease is a normal response to abnormal circumstances (Gabor Maté).

Common signs or conditions you might notice medically

- Diabetes
- High blood pressure
- Crushing chest pain
- Headaches that wake you up at night
- Physical body pain that isn't changing with movement
- Temperature/fevers
- Cancer
- Broken bones

- Rapid weight gain or loss without any change to lifestyle
- Intense pain

When is the best time to use it?

- You have been in a sudden severe accident.
- Sudden severe onset of symptoms.
- Pain or illness that isn't going away with rest.
- Pain that isn't changing with movement.
- You have a symptom that just doesn't seem right to you. Always trust your gut. (Not sure how to connect to your intuition? We'll get to that in Chapter 5).
- You have a chronic illness that is severe and needs medication or surgery to preserve your life.

Tools and guidance for this approach

- Find a medical doctor you trust and can have open conversations with.
- If you can't do the above, find another doctor.

How Do You Know if You're in the Space Between?

You've been told there's nothing wrong, yet you feel like your body isn't working quite right. *Or* you've been diagnosed with a condition, and the treatment options don't seem to address the underlying cause.

Remember, our bodies are always talking to us. The messages begin energetically, with subtle senses that we can often find hard to logically or consciously reason for. This doesn't mean they're invalid. When we don't address these subtle messages, dysfunction arises. This is a result of our bodies needing to adapt to the environment we continue to expose them to. Finally, when we've been ignoring or not addressing the under-lying cause of our symptoms, they get to the point where a threshold is hit and we're given a medical diagnosis, a label, drugs, or surgery for management.

Much like if you have type 2 diabetes. The kind that has reached the point where you need insulin to live. Working solely on the functional and energetic levels is dangerous, and it also makes it harder for you to heal. In the case of chronic symptoms that eventually turn into disease, using all the lenses is a great idea. Because even in this state, only using the medical lens will often keep you from dying, but it may not make you feel alive.[14]

There is a difference between not being dead and being alive.

MY OWN ENERGETIC WHISPERS

Understanding the kind of care your body needs is very close to my heart. Literally.

When I was around 4 years old, I remember telling Mum that I had chest pain when we were walking around our local lake. Being the incredibly smart, gorgeous woman she is, she knew that a 4-year-old complaining of chest pain was an abnormal thing, so she organized for me to have a host of different investigations, all of which came back clear.

In the subsequent years, I experienced chronic UTIs up until I was around halfway through primary school. I remember frequently doing at home tests for infections and having UTI medication to stop my wee from burning. Early high school was when I had the crushing chest pain and rapid heart rate incident on the beach, and the amazing doctors and nurses repaired the plumbing and electrical issues with my heart with multiple surgeries. But even after having the surgeries and fixing the structural issues, I would still get this crushing chest pain on occasion. So much so that, on a particular day, I ended up at the local GP's office, and, after a quick ECG, he told me I needed to go straight to the emergency department because my scan showed that I could be having a heart attack. Thankfully, after more investigation, that wasn't the case.

When I look back to that time and ask, *What was my body telling me?* I realized that I was incredibly stressed and had just had an argument with my older brother, Harrison. My chest pain wasn't being caused by something that needed medical attention; it was coming up because I wasn't saying what was on my chest. I wasn't "getting it off my chest."

～

The body will always tell you things in little energetic whispers first and if you don't pay attention, the whispers continue to get louder and louder and louder.

In the last year, that's what happened to me. I finally started to *really* listen to my body. Throughout my life, I've had what I thought were random intrusive memories or thoughts that "everyone has." Memories of me being sexually taken advantage of multiple times by an older man when I was around 4 years old. These memories would come in random flashes during the day and would always be in the same situations. It wasn't until I started doing the sexuality quarter of a personal development program I was a part of that the memories started to become more and more frequent. They came closer to the surface and no matter how much I still tried to ignore them or convince myself that "everyone" had these random thoughts, my body was ready to see them. My body finally felt safe enough to feel what was coming up. It started testing up on my kinesiology sessions, and my body wanted to release it. My skin was breaking out, and I started to develop a dry rash on my upper back. After doing some deep work with energetic practitioners and coaches and finding safety in my body to be able to hold all of my emotions, the physical manifestations of my subconscious patterns started to disappear.

When I look back, of course I started to get chest pain when I was 4. When you can't find the words at 4, your body tries to communicate it for you. I needed to get it off my chest. This same crushing chest pain would happen even after my surgeries when I wasn't expressing what I needed to at the time. From an energetic perspective, the UTIs and kidneys can be linked with fear, bad memories, allowing people to manipulate and control you, sexual pressure, and shame. It was no accident that I started to develop recurrent UTIs in early childhood.

Much like your aunt, your body can't keep a secret.

Your body will express it in ways that it thinks you can handle. As the famous author and trauma expert Dr. Bessel van der Kolk says, "Your body keeps the score."

This isn't to say that if you get chest pain, what occurred in my past happened in yours. But it is to say that your body is always talking to you. When we allow the things we can't see to stay in our bodies, they start to become what we can see, manifesting in physical body dysfunction and eventually in disease. When we avoid, ignore, put off, or gaslight ourselves into not acknowledging something that is true for ourselves, it doesn't go away. It manifests in different ways until we acknowledge and feel our way through it. It's like my little brother Jeremy's favorite book, *We're Going on a Bear Hunt,* implies: You can't go over it. You can't go under it. You have to go through it.

There's no one type of healthcare that's better than another. It's about matching the type of care with what your body needs at the time. For something like crushing chest pain, I needed to go to the hospital to make sure it wasn't a heart attack. But when I received the news that it wasn't, did that mean I was making the chest pain up? No! It just meant I needed to use a different lens. I needed to listen to what my body was telling me from a different perspective.

IT'S ALL ABOUT NUANCE, IT'S ALL ABOUT COLOR

We're always changing and adapting, and, just like people can outgrow each other, sometimes we need to look at and change what type of healthcare we're predominantly using. If you start experiencing a new symptom, it's like you're going back into the dating pool. We might dabble in all different kinds of people to see what works and what definitely doesn't. You can be left blaming yourself or blaming them, thinking that it's all in your head, when really… it just wasn't a good match.

**It's not about changing the healthcare system;
it's about changing the way we use the system.**

So, how do we know what type of help we need? Our bodies are leading the show.

We can read all of the most up-to-date research and health books, and we can know all of the "right" things to do, but our bodies are contextual. There can be a piece of advice that serves the majority of people the majority of the time, but sometimes it's not helpful for us.

Take fasting, for instance. Fasting and time restricted eating can be highly beneficial when done at the right time in our cycles and when our 4 Female Fundamentals are taken care of. However, if we aren't balanced in our Fundamentals, fasting can be perceived by the body as another stressor and can be counterintuitive.

It's not mainstream versus alternative. Drugs versus no drugs. Medicine versus Natural.

Your body wants the best of all worlds.
There is a place for everyone.
You just need to find your match.
The first step is always connecting to your body
and developing a deep trust with it.

So, we need to remember a few things:

1. No one type of healthcare modality or service is better than another. They all serve a purpose, and it's important to understand what type of care you need.
2. How you know what you need is by connecting with your body.

It's not black and white. The color is where the magic is.

Chapter 3

WHAT'S MY BODY TRYING TO TELL ME?

~

A question that's not as difficult to answer
as we might think.

YOUR WHOLE BODY IS A VITAL SIGN

You know that famous scene from *The Notebook?* The one where Ryan Gosling asks Rachel McAdams, "What do you want?" and she replies, "It's not that simple!" That's exactly the cluster fuck of what it can feel like when we begin to try and understand what our bodies are telling us. *What does my period pain mean? Why is my hair falling out? Why am I so tired all the time? Is it normal to wake up feeling anxious?*

Unfortunately, I can't teach you everything you need to know about how the body works in this chapter, or even this book, but, let me tell you, you don't actually need to know everything. All you need to know and understand is how to recognize when things are going well, when things are getting a little rocky, and when your body is screaming at you to reach out for help. We get into trouble when we don't understand the difference between these messages and they go by unchecked for too long.

UNDERSTANDING YOUR BODY'S MESSAGES IS AS SIMPLE AS DATING

When it comes to understanding our bodies' messages, we have green flags, beige flags, and red flags.

Green flags are signs that your body is LOVING you and is functioning exactly how it's meant to. It's like when your date can both poke fun at themselves and love themselves, when they care for you and also have boundaries, when they're emotionally intelligent, funny, and have a great group of friends.

Beige flags are signs that your body isn't loving what you're doing, but it can push through. They mean that what you're experiencing isn't life-threatening, but it's often unpleasant. They're warning signs of the potential for the situation to get worse in the future.

In dating, they're things that make you cringe a little but aren't a deal-breaker. Sort of like when you see the person you're dating pick their nose and eat it or put their hands down their pants to pick their wedgy. Not a deal breaker, perhaps, but not a comfortable thing to witness. In terms of your body, beige flags are little hints and whispers that things are off. The more of these that stack up, the more we head into red flag territory. Addressing your Female Fundamentals (Chapter 4) is how we move from beige to green flags.

Red flags from your body are signs that it's at the end of its ability to cope. It needs help to restore balance, and further investigation is needed because there could be something more serious going on. In dating, these are deal breakers—do not pass go and do not collect $200. Things like having the emotional maturity of a 9-year-old, taking you out for an expensive dinner and "forgetting" their wallet, spending the whole time talking about themselves, or having hyper-controlling behavior.

Sometimes some of us get a little color-blind and confuse red flags for beige or green flags, just like that one friend who always seems to date people who are walking red flags, and they get a shock when they finally realize how much of a dick they were. The same goes for our bodies. We can think things like diabetes, autoimmune conditions, and the need for thyroid medication pop up out of nowhere, because we've confused beige flags for green flags for too long.

So, how can we avoid the beige and red flags and be given the green flag from our bodies? We need to learn the language of the body and understand what we might be doing that could be turning us color-blind and allowing the beige or red flag patterns to continue and cause disease.

Remember:

Green flags = Signs your body is functioning well

Beige flags = Signs your body doesn't quite have what it needs

Red flags = Signs your body needs help now

THINGS THAT MIGHT BE TURNING YOU COLORBLIND...

It's society's running joke that women will rip your head off before their period or that our partners must go out and buy us chocolate to get on our good side. Ads for pain relief when we experience that little niggle of a headache. Thinking we need to be on birth control because all of our friends are. Often, the things that turn us color-blind are what we've accepted as normal in society. This would be perfect if we were all happy and healthy. But we're not. So, this colorblind thing isn't really working out for us. Like when you marry someone because you fell in love with their potential, not who they were. You fell in love with your delusion.

Whether we have or haven't been given an answer for our symptoms, it's important to not get attached...

WHAT'S YOUR HEALTH ATTACHMENT STYLE?

Like attachment styles in relationships, what I've come to realize is that people have an attachment style with their relationship to their own health. Attachment theory was originally developed by John Bowlby and Mary Ainsworth, and it explains our patterns of how we bond with another person.[15]

"Avoidants" tend to not trust others; "anxious" tend to trust others more than themselves, and "secure" have high self-trust and a balanced belief in others. I see these same patterns among patients, loved ones, and even myself when it comes to our relationships with health.

So, which one are you?

Avoidant Health Type

I like to think of avoidant people as purposefully "color blind." They trick themselves into thinking that the red and beige flags are green flags. They think their bodies are indestructible, often push themselves until their bodies whack them with a significant illness, and often don't trust others.

Common phrases of the avoidant health type
- "It's not that bad."
- "I'll push on."
- "Suzie next door has it worse than me."
- "I don't have time."
- "It's not worth the money."
- "I'll deal with it when I really need to."

- "I don't trust doctors."
- "I have a high pain threshold." (I once had a patient ask me to punch them to prove how high their pain threshold was… I think it's fair to say they had some avoidant tendencies).

Common behaviors

- Difficulty sitting in emotional discomfort, even when it's slight discomfort.
- Ignoring symptoms of the body, or covering them up with substances.
- Putting others before themselves.
- Always on the move.
- Often rely on numbing behaviors like binge watching TV, binge eating, consuming alcohol at the end of the day (or sometimes the start), and struggle to sit in boredom.
- Fear of being seen as lazy if they rest.
- Notice symptoms and want to shut them down, either by ignoring them or taking something to cover them up.
- Intellectualize and gaslight themselves into believing their symptoms aren't a big deal.

How it feels in your body

- Numb "stable"
- Heavy
- Dull
- Often a lot of energy in the head
- Difficult to feel or notice at all

Impacts of this type

They often allow small dysfunctions to build into larger, more serious conditions, resulting in chronic illness.

When we're avoidant, our functional health starts to deteriorate, and then physical manifestations can appear. We can have irregular bowel habits or menstrual cycles, pains, rashes, acne, or stretch marks, headaches, and so on. It's not life-threatening, but our bodies are telling us to pay attention and change something. We might continue to ignore these signs, and our physical symptoms get worse, until eventually our bodies scream out for help in the form of a disease that we need medication or surgery for. And even then, sometimes we continue to ignore our bodies.

Ways you can move to a more secure type

Understand the difference between green, beige, and red flags. Purposefully connect to your body every day. Remember, you and your body are on the same team, and you should aim to respond to those niggles and feelings by first acknowledging them.

Anxious Health Type

People with anxious attachment to their bodies often want to know every piece of information and are continuously on the hunt for every new thing that promises to be the magical fix. The bottom line—they fear that no matter how much they do, eventually something bad will happen with their health. They don't trust their bodies.

Common phrases of the anxious health type

- "I used to be vegetarian, but now I'm a full carnivore."
- "Do you have any new health podcast recommendations, I've listened to them all."
- "I pretty much have my doctor's number on speed dial."
- "Is that flutter in my neck a blood vessel problem?"
- "I'm doing daily breathwork, ice baths, saunas, lifting weights, getting my protein, removing all my toxins. What else should I be doing?"
- "I feel like no matter how much I do, my body will fail me."

Common behaviors

- Googling every symptom
- Hyperfixating on getting everything perfect with their bodies
- Looking at their health stats on their fitness device multiple times per day
- Constant hygiene practices
- Health fad queens
- Overly concerned with physical appearance

How it feels in your body

- Ungrounded
- Panicked
- Rushed
- Worry
- Rumination
- Fear

Impacts of this type

They often feel highly stressed and spend a lot of energy trying to find the magic fix outside of themselves, never feeling satisfied with their health. The concern that something will eventually "get them" consumes their thoughts, and they often have difficulty relaxing with their bodies. They may also feel guilt around missing a workout class or having a "flexi day" with their diets.

Ways you can move to a more secure type

Remember, your body is extremely resilient. It's been keeping you alive without you consciously having to remind it to. Understand the difference between green, beige, and red flags. Purposefully ground into your body.

You'll notice I say "connect to your body" for avoidant types and "ground into your body" for anxious types. This is because avoidants need to build the awareness of their bodies, and anxious types need to build the trust in their bodies.

Anxious-Avoidant Health Type

Anxious-avoidant types listen to their bodies and often seek practitioners, such as naturopaths, Chinese medicine doctors, medical doctors, chiropractors, and kinesiologists, for help but don't get the results they want. Consequently, they feel disheartened and frustrated, swapping between not trusting others and being annoyed at their bodies. They've spent so much time and energy searching for answers that they're giving up on ever finding them.

Common phrases of the anxious/avoidant health type

- "That was a waste of time."
- "(Insert health profession) is a waste of money."
- "I may as well not try."
- "My body is going to break down anyway."
- "(Insert health modality or trend) helped for a little while."

Common behaviors

- Seeking help and expecting instant results
- "Doctor shopping"
- Jumping on health trends
- A draw full of half-used supplements and medications

How it feels in your body

- Confusion
- Frustration
- Anger
- Out of control
- Hopeless
- Like a roller-coaster

Impacts of this type

They often develop a simultaneous distrust in themselves and in health practitioners. This can result in not seeking help when needed.

Ways you can move to a more secure type

Understand the difference between green, beige, and red flags. Purposefully connect and ground into your body every day. Lasting change happens over time, so find something that makes sense for you and give it a go for at least three months. Remember, your body and you are on the same team.

Secure Health Type

When we know that the body is inherently always supporting and loving us, when we know what our bodies fundamentally need to function at their best, when we know and trust in our own abilities, we assume responsibility for our health and life. This ultimately gives us freedom and safety in our bodies. We know that when we experience symptoms, it's just how our bodies communicate with us. We know how to support our bodies. We know what type of support we might need to reach out for. We know our bodies aren't as fragile as we might think. We know we aren't broken if everything isn't perfect.

Defining characteristic: secure types trust that their bodies know exactly what to do, and they trust themselves to know when they need to change something or reach out for help.

Common phrases of the secure type

- "I've noticed that this new thing has started happening with my body. I'll see if it settles, otherwise I'll get it checked."
- "I know when I change (X part of my lifestyle), my body will feel like its healthy self again."

- "This is really out of the ordinary for me. I'm going to book in with (X practitioner)."

Common behaviors

- Regularly connecting to their bodies
- Seeking help
- Tuning into and giving their bodies what they need
- Knowing when things are urgent and when they're not
- Health is important to them but doesn't consume their lives

How it feels in your body

- Calm
- Grounded
- Certain

What attachment style resonates with you the most?

We shift to a secure attachment more readily when we understand and believe that our bodies are always looking after us. This understanding comes with basic knowledge and the ability to tune into our bodies, and responding appropriately to the signals using the green, beige, and red flag system. This gives us the confidence to know when we can change things ourselves and when we need to reach out for help.

HOW DO WE CATCH THE SIGNS BEFORE THEY TURN INTO RED FLAGS?

The most basic way we can tell if our bodies are doing OK, or not, is through our vital signs: breathing, heart rate, temperature, and blood pressure. When we experience changes in these signs, it often means something significant is happening. An infection, heart attack, blood clot, burst lung, internal bleeding. When we think of how our bodies talk to us, we often think in terms of these vital signs. We use the term "vital" here to mean something that is essential for life. When one or many of these vital signs are abnormal, we know the body is under significant distress.

We also use health screenings to know if our bodies are healthy or not. We get those "fun" but necessary regular skin checks, cervical screening tests (pap smears), and bowel and breast cancer screenings. These behavioral changes have saved many lives and are necessary, but what if we could listen to even more subtle messages from the body? What if we didn't see vital signs as markers for if we were living or dying, but markers for how alive we felt?

Being not dead isn't the same as being alive.

Waiting for one of our main four vital signs or a health screening test to show something abnormal is like waiting for your final year report card at school and not receiving any feedback on your grades throughout the year. Hoping that everything turns out OK at the end of the year is a backwards way of thinking if our goal is to have thriving health (or grades). If we had gotten feedback throughout the year, we could have made changes along the way, making it a hell of a lot easier by removing stress and avoiding the feeling of limbo.

The way we do this for our bodies is by understanding that the whole body is a vital sign. In recent years, our menstrual cycle has been coined as the fifth vital sign. What many of us don't realize is that things like our skin, nails, hair, tongue, gut, mental state, sleep, and energy are also vital(ity) signs. The small symptoms, like dandruff, waking in the night, and weight gain, are telling us something—that there is an imbalance between the resources of the internal body and the demand of the external world.

Now, you might be thinking, *That's why I wear my health tech device. It gives me live feedback on things like my sleep, heart rate variability, ovulation, and step count.* Having a device that gives you more specific data is amazing; it often points us in the right direction, but we're still left trying to figure out what we need to change to get the data looking better.

HEALTH TECH CAN COMPLEMENT OUR BODIES' NATURAL COMMUNICATION CHANNELS

Let me tell you a story of Isobel. She's super into her fitness and competes in national competitions. She originally came to see me because she was experiencing fatigue, dizziness, a foggy head, and troubles with her weight. She mentioned that, even after her blood tests came back clear, her health data always showed that she rarely dropped into a restful sleep zone. She had changed her sleep routine and was diligent about the usual culprits—blue light, sunlight, caffeine, and room temperature. Even still, her health data didn't change. The data was great at telling her what wasn't working for her body, but why it was happening was left for her to figure out. Based on her symptoms, it was clear that there was something going on under the surface.

After we assessed her by addressing her 4 Female Fundamentals (which you'll learn about in the next chapter), it was clear that we needed to support all four of her Fundamentals. We altered the order and timing of her food, gave her specific supplementation for nutritional imbalances that had resulted from previous high stress, and incorporated some lifestyle changes to support her nervous system and metabolism. After two weeks of the changes, she could feel that her head was clear, her energy had boosted, she was stronger in the gym, and was waking up to her alarm not thinking that she could use another full day of sleep. She noticed that her sleep data on her device had changed too.

The good news is that when we become attuned to our bodies, we realize our sleep, skin, energy levels, menstrual cycle, hair growth or loss, our tongue and our mental state can tell us why we're experiencing symptoms like fatigue, poor sleep, period pain, and IBS. When we understand how they speak to us, we understand *why* we're experiencing our symptoms and can address the root cause.

Think of your vital signs as a scale. They can be slight, almost like telepathy. Like when you ask someone's advice about something, but you know deep down what you already need to do. You might be wondering if you should take that new job, tell your toxic partner it's over, or buy that new outfit. We know the answer. When we feel anxious, happy, or guilty, these emotions are all telling us something.

The signs for vitality can get a little louder, often manifesting physically, for example, in the form of a painful shorter period, worse PMS, stretch marks, acne, bloating, or trouble sleeping. Eventually, the signs can get a little louder again when things like blood tests and scans show there's more significant adaptation happening in our bodies. When we're under significant load, the other typical four main vital signs will be our final warning.

Because of this, the one thing I believe without a shadow of a doubt is that your body is gifting you your symptoms. Your whole body is a vital sign. Let's take a peek at what it might be telling you...

**You can tell a lot from the body
when you learn to listen to it.**

～～

Let's make navigating what your body is telling you super easy.

Remember... all of these symptoms are messages from your body. They mean two things: your body is either balancing or not balancing your internal resources with the external demand *and* they're showing you the way forward.

MENSTRUAL CYCLE

In recent years, the menstrual cycle has been coined the fifth vital sign, and for good reason. It provides a direct insight into how our hormones are functioning across the whole month. Our hormones are a window into how our bodies are maintaining overall balance. Don't just stop there.

When we understand, for example, that the symptom of heavy periods may be due to high estrogen, we can take it a step further and continue to ask why our estrogen is high. From my experience, when we continue to ask why, it always comes back to the 4 Female Fundamentals.

The menstrual cycle is a marker of fertility, but it's also so much more than that. Regardless of whether you ever have a baby, the hormonal and rhythmic shifts that occur across a woman's month and lifetime allow for greater bone, heart, gut, and brain health. The monthly bleed also functions to detoxify the body and connect to the flow of life. The womb is associated with the sacral chakra, connecting each woman to creativity, transformation, and pleasure.

Green Flags (signs your body is doing its thang!):

The following are for women not on hormonal contraceptives. Taking external hormones affects the natural flow and rhythm of natural hormone production.

- **Regular menstrual cycle (for reproductive-age women).** This means from day one to the next day one. For ovulation to occur, the cycle needs to be between 21–35 days. Ideally, closer to 28 days. The length ideally stays within a 0–2-day difference each month.
- **Pain free**. At most, you may feel a four-day old bruise level of sensitivity. The pain shouldn't be hindering your day or life.
- **3–7 days of bleeding.** Good level of estrogen in your body.
- **Clots no bigger than an Australian 5-cent piece (or a US nickel).** Healthy levels of estrogen and inflammation.
- **Primarily cherry red in color.** Healthy turnover of the endometrial lining. Good levels of hormones and iron.
- **Changes in cervical mucus throughout the cycle.** White paste builds in amount, swapping to thin and clear mucus mid cycle, then changing to a thicker white, becoming dry and less copious.
- **Increased hunger after ovulation**. Progesterone release increases our metabolic rate; therefore, our demand for calories increases (by about 200 calories per day).[16]
- **Slight mood changes.** The large majority of our body's cells are sensitive to our hormones. With their natural ebb and flow across the month and

our lifespan, mood changes occur. If they are more significant and start to impact your relationships, then this is a beige flag.

The combination of all of these factors indicates a healthy menstrual cycle and that probable ovulation has occurred.

Beige Flags (the stuff we sometimes think of as healthy because it's common; it often won't kill you, but it's your body giving you a hint that it doesn't quite have the balance it needs):

- **Pain.** High prostaglandins (inflammation).
- **PMS/PMDD.** Copper and zinc imbalance. Watch your blood sugars and stress levels too.
- **Bloating.** Low sodium and potassium due to prolonged stress causing fluid to retain in tissues. Low stomach acid, which allows gas-producing bacteria to flourish.
- **Period poops (sloppy poos before and during period).** High prostaglandins in the body, usually due to a low level of magnesium and B6, inflammatory foods, and high levels of stress.
- **Clots larger than an Australian 10-cent piece (or a US quarter).** High estrogen.
- **Needing to change a tampon more often than every two hours.** High estrogen.
- **Needing to wear "double protection" (for example, a tampon and pad).** High estrogen.

- **Bleeding less than 3 days or more than 7 days.** Too little estrogen or too much estrogen, respectively.
- **Bleeding every two weeks.** Low progesterone due to absent or ineffective ovulation.
- **Brown spotting at the start or the end.** Old uterine lining from previous cycle, low progesterone, and altered estrogen.
- **Dark plum red color.** High estrogen, copper and iron imbalance.
- **Regular irregularity.** Periods that change in length every cycle but are generally between 21–35 days. Ovarian reserve may be affected.
- **Irregularity.** You're not ovulating consistently. Brain and ovary connections are affected. As with all of the above, look at your 4 Female Fundamentals.

Red Flags (it's time to seek further medical advice):
- **Bleeding during penetrative sex.** Depending on your age, body weight, and sex hormone levels, this could indicate low levels of estrogen and a fragile vaginal lining, or a growth or damage to the cervix.
- **Bleeding 12 months after final menstrual cycle.** Could indicate possible cancerous lesions.
- **Feeling of fullness in the lower abdomen area with pain down the legs.** Possible growth on the uterus, ovaries, or bowel.

- **Flooding.** High estrogen could be causing uterine fibroids. Flooding causes too much blood loss and can result in severe iron and oxygenation issues.
- **Loss of period for more than three months (unless you're in the perimenopause or menopausal age bracket).** Can indicate pregnancy or a problem with the brain or ovary, or the connection between the two.
- **Failure to begin the first menstrual cycle before 16 years old.** May indicate sex organ, brain, or genetic issue.
- **Pubic hair or breast budding before 8 years old.** Hormone levels high, which could be due to an endocrine organ problem or environmental exposure.

For any changes that you feel are out of the ordinary for you and raise concern, always seek assistance.

If you've been diagnosed with a condition or experience symptoms associated with your menstrual cycle, you'll find links to more information, including complete breakdowns, in the "Resources" section at the back of the book.

~

FERTILITY

Fertility is essential for the continuation of the human race, but nonessential to our current lives. Often, when our bodies are struggling to keep up basic functions, we may begin to notice changes in our menstrual cycles and troubles with fertility.

Green Flags

- **Consistently regular natural periods (without hormonal contraception).**
- **Mucous changes across the month.**

Beige Flags

- **Irregular periods.** Indicate irregular ovulation.
- **Failure to conceive after six months** of unprotected, ovulation-timed intercourse. Consider possible ovulation, sperm, or pathway blockage issues.
- **Frequent illness.** Immune system is crucial for health and can often struggle when basic functions of the body aren't being met, just like fertility.
- **Lack of mucus changes.** Possible insufficient ovulation.
- **Recurrent miscarriage.** Can frequently indicate insufficient progesterone levels.

Red Flags

- **Failure to conceive after 12 months** of unprotected, ovulation-timed, intercourse.
- **Bleeding during pregnancy.**
- **Losing more than 5 percent of prepregnancy weight from continual morning sickness.**

For any changes that you feel are out of the ordinary for you and raise concern, always seek assistance.

If you've been diagnosed with a condition or experience symptoms associated with fertility and pregnancy, you'll find links to more information, including complete breakdowns, in the "Resources" section at the back of the book.

~~~

GUT

The gut is how we break down and absorb nutrients to create life-sustaining substances in our bodies. It also provides a physical barrier to the outside world and, as such, is involved intimately with the immune system. Gut function is as much about what you're putting into your body as it is about getting the internal signal to function. The gut gives a clear window into how the fundamental aspects of the body are working.

Green Flags
- **Doing a poop at least once every day, sometimes even twice or three times.**
- **Wake up without bloating.**
- **Poop looks like a log or a chocolate bar.**
- **It sinks.**
- **Effortless to use bowels.**

Beige Flags

- **Feeling sick after you eat.** Gut inflammation (or was that chicken in fact past its use-by date?).
- **Bloating when you wake.** Stomach acid and enzymes low.
- **Farting and burping a lot after food.** Stomach acid low.
- **Bloating after you eat.** Pancreatic enzymes low.
- **Floating poop.** Trouble digesting fats.
- **Cycling between constipation and diarrhea.** Most likely underlying constipation.
- **Skipping a day or more between poops.** Slow metabolic rate and thyroid imbalance.
- **The need to strain.** Slowed gut motility due to Female Fundamental imbalance.
- **Going less than once a day.** Poor detox pathways.
- **Pebble like stool or loose stool.** Constipation, slowed gut motility, hypothyroid, mineral imbalance, dysregulated nervous system, inflammation.

Supporting your 4 Female Fundamentals is how to move your beige flags to green flags. Always

Red Flags

- **Sudden intense stomach pain.**
- **Blood in your poop.** Bleeding in lower gut (hemorrhoids, polyps, and so on).

- **Black poop.** Possible bleeding in upper gut.
- **Green, frothy, mucousy poop.** Parasites, gut infection.
- **Loss of bowel control.** Issue with spinal cord, pelvic floor muscles, or brain function.

For any changes that you feel are out of the ordinary for you and raise concern, always seek assistance.

If you've been diagnosed with a condition or experience symptoms associated with the gut, you'll find links to more information, including complete breakdowns, in the "Resources" section at the back of the book.

~~

SLEEP AND ENERGY

You don't have to read 500 research articles to know the benefits of sleep. We know that if we haven't had a good night's sleep, we're exactly like a toddler who missed their nap. We're crankier; we want sugar; if you look at us the wrong way, we'll snap, and we can't think clearly, deliriously muddling our way through the day. Unlike eating well or moving well, sleep is passive. You can't actively choose to fall asleep, even when you've set up the perfect bedtime routine. Ultimately, it's our bodies passively choosing that sends us to sleep. Sleep, therefore, is a symptom of the balance between our internal bodily resources and our external environment.

Green Flags

- **Feeling resilient when change happens.**
- **Energy when you wake up and sustained throughout the day.**
- **Fall asleep between 5–15 minutes.**
- **Sleep through the night majority of nights** (unless you're older than 50). Waking to use the toilet once may be considered normal in the absence of other symptoms.
- **Consistency in your routine.**

Beige Flags

- **Taking longer than 15 minutes to fall asleep.** Active stress levels (high cortisol), low calcium levels, low melatonin levels.
- **Taking less than two minutes to fall asleep.** Exhaustion, sleep apnea.
- **Falling asleep as soon as your head hits the pillow.** Exhaustion, blood sugars, sleep apnea.
- **Falling asleep as soon as you sit down.** Sleep apnea, exhaustion.
- **Feeling tired in the afternoon.** Blood sugars and stress not regulated across the day.
- **Waking up every 2–3hrs.** High cortisol levels, low magnesium.
- **Needing to get up frequently through the night to wee.** Structural—prostate (men), prolapse (women).

Functional—insulin resistance, adrenal exhaustion, and poor salt-fluid balance.

- **Waking up tired.** Prolonged adrenal use, thyroid dysfunction, low iron.
- **The need for naps.** Iron deficiency, sugar crash, circadian rhythm disrupted.

Red Flags

- **Feeling breathless when you walk up a flight of stairs**. Poor oxygen, with causes ranging from low iron to poor lung and heart function.
- **Feeling fatigued and noticing weight loss without active effort.**
- **Fatigue with fevers.**
- **Fatigue not relieved by rest.**
- **Fatigue with body pain that doesn't change with movement.**

For any changes that you feel are out of the ordinary for you and raise concern, always seek assistance.

If you've been diagnosed with a condition or experience symptoms associated with sleep and energy, you'll find links to more information, including complete breakdowns, in the "Resources" section at the back of the book.

~~~

HAIR

Hair helps to provide insulation and temperature control particularly on our heads and bodies. The hair in the nose and ears helps to support our immune systems. Where our hair grows or doesn't grow, and its texture and pigment, can give us insight into what's happening inside our bodies, from hormone imbalance to cardiovascular disease.

Green Flags

- **Thick, strong head hair.**
- **Minimal dark or coarse facial hair (exception if this is genetic and based on heritage).**

Beige Flags

- **Noticing loose hair strands in the bed when you wake up.** Hormonal change (this can be normal if postpartum or menopause), gut malabsorption, poor protein intake, iron or copper deficiency.
- **Thinning outside of your eyebrows.** Underfunctioning thyroid.
- **Widening of your middle part.** High androgens (male characteristic hormones like testosterone), nutrient deficiency or malabsorption.
- **Circular patch of head hair not growing.** Protein, iron, zinc, copper, or B7 deficiency. Consider autoimmunity, which can be addressed by reducing inflammation and supporting stress levels. Ultimately,

as with all beige flags, take care of your Female Fundamentals (Chapter 4).

- **Hair thinning.** Need more protein, zinc, selenium. Could be a sign of hypothyroid or anemia.
- **Dandruff.** Lack of essential fatty acids or zinc.
- **Early graying.** Lack of protein, copper excess, zinc deficiency, lack of vitamin B7 and B12.
- **Dry hair.** Essential fatty acids low.
- **Receding hairline (on women).** Higher levels of a subtype of testosterone called DHT. This often also causes jawline acne and darker facial and body hair.
- **Facial hair.** In women, this indicates high androgens.

Red Flags

- **Losing hair growth on lower limbs, along with tight skin.** Diabetes and cardiovascular risk.

For any changes that you feel are out of the ordinary for you and raise concern, always seek assistance.

If you've been diagnosed with a condition or experience symptoms associated with your hair, you'll find links to more information, including complete breakdowns, in the "Resources" section at the back of the book.

SKIN

Our skin forms a boundary for our bodies, helping to let "friends" in and keep "foes" out.

It's a large component of our immune and detoxification systems. It's equally important to consider what we put on our skin as it is to consider what the appearance of our skin is telling us about what's happening under the surface.

Green Flags

- Clear skin that's elastic and strong.

Beige Flags

- **Stretch marks.** White stretch marks—relative zinc deficiency. Purple stretch marks—absolute zinc deficiency.
- **Acne.** Detox pathways need support.
- **Dry, itchy skin.** Deficiency of essential fatty acids, zinc, vitamin A, B, and C.
- **Easy to bruise.** Vitamin C and copper imbalance. Could also be a medication side effect.
- **Poor circulation.** Thyroid, metabolism, or oxygenation issues.
- **Always sweaty palms and feet.** Dysregulated nervous system.
- **Small red bumps on the back of your arms (chicken skin).** Vitamin A and zinc deficiency.
- **Skin tags.** Insulin resistance.

- **Skin discoloration in creases of neck, knees, armpits.** Excess blood glucose. Excess B3 (niacin).

Red Flags

- **Rash with small pustules in a line pattern**, often associated with burning pain.
- **Mole with a completely black component.**
- **Mole that has changed in shape or color or size.**
- **Rash accompanied by a fever.**

For any changes that you feel are out of the ordinary for you and raise concern, always seek assistance.

If you've been diagnosed with a condition or experience symptoms associated with your skin, you'll find links to more information, including complete breakdowns, in the "Resources" section at the back of the book.

~~~

NAILS

Nails are necessary for survival because they help us to scratch and itch. They help to remove potential threats from our skin as well as move swelling around the external layers. The health of your nails gives you a glimpse into the last 4–6 months of your health due to their typical growth rate.

Green Flags

- **Difficult to bend.**
- **Healthy cuticles.**
- **Smooth texture.**

Beige Flags

- **Bending weak nails.** Underfunctioning thyroid, poor nutrition.
- **Frayed cuticles.** Low essential fatty acids, calcium, and zinc. Possible malabsorption or hypothyroidism.
- **White spots on the nails.** It could be from physically whacking your nail or if it's on numerous nails, typically a sign of copper excess or zinc deficiency. Often associated with anxious or depressive mind frames due to the role zinc and copper play in creating neurotransmitters.
- **Spooned nails.** If you were to drop a droplet of water on the nail, it would sit there. This can be a sign of protein, iron, chromium, copper, or zinc deficiency.

Red Flags

- **Clubbed fingernails.** Poor circulation.
- **Blue or purple nail bed.** Poor oxygenation.

For any changes that you feel are out of the ordinary for you and raise concern, always seek assistance.

If you've been diagnosed with a condition or experience symptoms associated with your nails, you'll find links to more information, including complete breakdowns, in the "Resources" section at the back of the book.

~~~

TONGUE AND MOUTH

In many ways, your tongue and mouth are the window into your whole body. Often, when we're experiencing mouth and tongue issues, they're mimicked in our guts, and they're both extensions of each other.

Chinese medicine uses the tongue to understand how your different organs are functioning. The tongue is one of the few internal organs we can see. Knowing what it's telling us can give us a window into our overall function.

Green Flags

- Pink in color (not pale or red).
- Minimal cracking.
- No pain.
- Appears smooth, with some texture.
- No white or discoloration of the coating.
- Strong teeth.
- Odorless breath.

Beige Flags

- **Color.** Pale gums and tongue could mean iron deficiency, White coating—fungal overgrowth in the gut. Red tongue or gums—low vitamin C, high copper, elevated inflammation.
- **Texture.** Cracks down the center could mean gut inflammation, and low stomach acid and pancreatic enzymes.
- **Size.** An enlarged tongue, recognizable by a "wavy" shape on the sides, indicates possible sleep apnea, insulin resistance, or food allergies.
- **Sensation.** Burning mouth—iron and B vitamin deficiency, high stress.
- **Odor.** Bacterial overgrowth in gut, tooth decay or infection.
- **Bleeding gums.** Not enough vitamin C or too much copper.
- **Cracked lips and corner of mouth.** Malnutrition—B vitamins, vitamin C, zinc, iron.
- **Craving eating nonfoods (dirt, dry wall, soap).** Nutrient deficiency.

Red Flags

- **Purple-colored.** Poor oxygenation, lung and heart capacity.
- **Rash in or around mouth, accompanied by fever.**

For any changes that you feel are out of the ordinary for you and raise concern, always seek assistance.

If you've been diagnosed with a condition or experience symptoms associated with your tongue or mouth, you'll find links to more information, including complete breakdowns, in the "Resources" section at the back of the book.

~~~

VULVA, SEXUAL AND REPRODUCTIVE ORGANS

A quick anatomy lesson for those of you who think the vulva is mispronouncing the "Volvo" car. You can think of it like a house. The vulva is like the external appearance (everyone has a different one) made up of the external sexual and reproductive organs of a female body. It's what people have largely considered the vagina. The vagina is the entrance way; the cervix is the door; the uterus is the inside of the house, and the ovaries control how many people live in the house. They all play an important role, not only in reproduction but also in immunity, hormone production, brain development, bone strength, heart health, and gut health.

Energetically, it's where the creation of life takes place—the life of another and the sustained aliveness of our bodies. When there's a perceived threat to our lives or future lives, or we're over-giving to others and neglecting ourselves, or we feel ungrounded in our lives, often we can experience symptoms in these areas of our bodies. What might your body be telling you?

Green Flags

- **Pain-free sex.**
- **Moist, supple tissue.**
- **Neutral smell.**
- **Ability to expand and contract.**

Beige Flags

- **Painful sex.** Vaginismus, cysts, endometriosis, adenomyosis.
- **Bleeding during sex (not associated with menstrual cycle).** Cervical cyst, lack of estrogen, vaginismus.
- **Itching.** Infection, low estrogen.
- **Cottage cheese discharge.** Yeast infection.

Note: Some STIs, like chlamydia, are largely asymptomatic in women.

Red Flags

- **Fish-like smell.** Sign of bacterial vaginosis infection.
- **Green discharge and fever.** Infection.
- **Bleeding in menopause 12 months after final period.** Possible cancerous lesion.
- **Dull ache in lower abdomen,** with pain down your leg or into your hips.

For any changes that you feel are out of the ordinary for you and raise concern, always seek assistance.

If you've been diagnosed with a condition or experience symptoms associated with your vulva, sexual and reproductive organs, you'll find links to more information, including complete breakdowns, in the "Resources" section at the back of the book.

~~~

IMMUNE SYSTEM

Our immune systems are what differentiate self from others. What is *my* tissue and what is *something else* that is invading or abnormal to us. It's the physical and chemical boundary of the body. Physically, your skin, gut and sinuses and chemically, multiple layers that begin in your blood and mucus membranes.

You can think of it like the different levels of law enforcement. In the case of autoimmune conditions, it's like people calling the cops on themselves—your body has confused self for others.

Green Flags
- **Recover from sickness easily and quickly.**
- **Healthy gut function.** Refer to gut section above.
- **Healthy skin.** Refer to skin section above.

Beige Flags
- **Recurrent infections.**
- **Infections of different types at the same time.**
- **Getting sick any time "there's something going around."**

- **Skin and gut troubles.** Refer to previous respective sections.
- **Seasonal allergies.**

Red Flags
- **Diagnosed with autoimmune disease.**
- **Can't recover from mild sickness without outside help.**
- **Anaphylaxis.**

For any changes that you feel are out of the ordinary for you and raise concern, always seek assistance.

If you've been diagnosed with a condition or experience symptoms associated with the immune system, you'll find links to more information, including complete breakdowns, in the "Resources" section at the back of the book.

~~

MENTAL HEALTH

Our mental health is how our bodies balance our beliefs, social connections, and emotions to handle external stressors and facilitate connections with others, ultimately making decisions that are in alignment with our survival and the wellbeing of others.

Like all other aspects of our bodies, mental health isn't the absence of disease but an ability to achieve balance in all aspects of our lives. That balance is between our bodies' raw materials and the perceived demands of our external world. As we know, altering our internal environment with things like alcohol can change our behavior and emotions, and having a lack of sleep can make us more cranky than usual. Your mental state is determined by both your internal resources and your external environment.

Green Flags

- **Feeling a range of emotions throughout the day.**
- **Ability to self soothe and regulate.**
- **Capacity for empathy.**
- **Strong connection with others.**
- **Capacity for vulnerability.**
- **Ability to connect to the 8 C's** of self-compassion, curiosity, clarity, creativity, calm, confidence, courage, and connectedness.

Beige Flags

- **Not feeling safe to express or feel emotions.**
- **Inability to sit still.**
- **Feeling unsettled in calm environments.**
- **Hyperaggressive behavior.**
- **Over intellectualizing.**
- **Wake up anxious.**
- **Wake up angry.**
- **Confusion.**
- **Difficulty making decisions.**

There is a wide array of nutrient discrepancies and hormonal changes that can contribute to conditions like dyslexia, ADHD, anxiety, and depression. Remember, these adaptations in behavior and thought patterns are often healthy responses to abnormal internal or external environments. Supporting your body in both the internal and external aspects can be transformational.

Red Flags

- **Suicidal thoughts.**
- **Displeasure for things that you used to find pleasurable.**
- **Exhaustion—mentally and physically.**
- **Withdrawal.**
- **Personality changes**—drug abuse, brain lesion, infection.

If you are having suicidal thoughts, please contact your country's local mental health resource.

For any changes that you feel are out of the ordinary for you and raise concern, always seek assistance.

If you've been diagnosed with a condition or experience symptoms associated with mental health, you'll find links to more information, including complete breakdowns, in the "Resources" section at the back of the book.

GENERAL

Across your entire body's functions, there are general patterns you can look out for in order to know whether your body is telling you it has everything it needs or it wants you to change something.

Green Flags

- **Rhythm**. Your menstrual cycle is regular; your bowel habits are regular; you digest food well, and your skin is clear.
- **Adaptability**. The ability to adapt is the ability to survive.

Beige Flags

- **Lumps under armpits or in your groin.**
- **Painful periods.**
- **Irregular periods**
- **Bowel movements less than once a day or more than three times a day.**
- **Frequent sickness.**
- **Lack of energy upon waking.**
- **Waking during the night.**

Red Flags (general signs and symptoms that mean you should speak to your doctor):

This is not a complete and exhaustive list. If you're concerned about any symptoms, speak to your doctor.

- **Rapid weight gain or weight loss** without any active change to diet or lifestyle.
- **Pain or headaches that wake you at night.**
- **New onset of symptoms that concern you.**
- **A symptom that affects your ability to function.**
- **Loss or change in menstrual cycle across three months.**
- **Night sweats.**
- **Diffuse lower abdominal pain with a feeling of fullness.**
- **Lost your period.** This could be a green flag if you're menopausal or wanting to fall pregnant.
- **Sweating through your clothes at night.**
- **Blood in stool or black stool.**
- **Any body pain that doesn't change with movement.** Chest pain, lower abdominal pain and so on...
- **Inability to control bowel or bladder.**

If you find yourself at any stage after reading the criteria for the conditions thinking, *That's me, that's what I have,* catch yourself and ask, *Why is my body experiencing this? What is it trying to tell me?* Start to become more concerned with the why than you are with the what. If you don't have red flags, head straight for balancing your Female Fundamentals. If you do have red flags, see your practitioner. Remember, it's not an accident that your body is responding like this. They're having a healthy response to an abnormal environment.

Your diagnosis
isn't the destination.

"WHY?"—THE CRITICAL QUESTION

When a patient comes to me and says, "I have PCOS, anxiety, and anemia," I often find myself thinking, *Yeh, but why?* Telling me "what" you have doesn't tell me why you have it.

The role of a diagnosis is to make it a hell of a lot easier to talk about what we're experiencing. Imagine a world where we didn't have them...

"So, I have these red, inflamed spots on my skin that sometimes have pus coming out of them, and they seem to come out more around my jawline when I'm about to get my period."

"Oh, so you have hormonal acne."

"I have heavy periods that are often painful and cause nausea. I notice I have pain when I try to poop and sometimes even pain when I have sex. I had surgery, and they found excess tissue on the outside of my organs."

"Oh, so you have endometriosis."

"I seem to be experiencing a lot of pain in my arm after I fell off my skateboard, and my wrist looks disfigured now."

"Oh, so you have a broken arm."

If you have been diagnosed with hormonal acne, endometriosis, or even a broken arm, this isn't to discount the diagnosis—it's to get you to start questioning why your body is deciding to respond this way.

~

Let me Show you What I Mean...

I recently started seeing a patient, let's call her Lisa. She's in her mid 30s and had suffered from her first grand mal seizure only a couple of months prior. She had been to see a neurologist, who excluded a brain tumor or aneurysm from being the cause for her sudden seizures. After the investigations, she was diagnosed with nongenetic epilepsy of unknown origin and prescribed a drug.

After a couple of weeks on the drug, she noticed she was feeling better. Less foggy in the head and fewer episodes of the "pre-epileptic fit feeling," as she described it. She mentioned, "I *do* have epilepsy, the doctor diagnosed me, and the medication is working."

This whole scenario convinced Lisa that she had epilepsy because the drug made her feel better and if she stopped taking the drug, she may experience another episode. This is the reality for many people, whether they've been diagnosed with PCOS and the pill has made their periods "regular" or the SSRIs have aided to relieve their anxiety.

What if the medication was giving her body exactly what it was trying to tell her it needed? What if we used it as a diagnostic tool instead of a therapeutic one? The medication she was given helped to rebalance the salt in her brain, which helped to slow the nerve impulses and control her neurological function. What I didn't tell you about Lisa was that prior to her first seizure, she, a single parent, had been working three jobs, and, in her words, was "severely burned out."

When our bodies are under chronic, severe stress, they crave salt because we need a balance of sodium, potassium, and magnesium to create our stress hormones. Having this context, what do you think her seizures were trying to tell her? Could it be that the seizures were telling her that her internal body didn't have enough raw materials to keep up with the demand she was putting on herself? Based on the timeline of her history and the fact that her brain scans were clear of tumors, aneurysms, or anything abnormal in the structure of her brain, I'd say her body was giving her a wake-up call. A gift, albeit scary, but necessary if she wanted to continue living.

DOES THIS MEAN WE DON'T TAKE THE MEDICATION?

No, not at all. It means we stop, pause, and think. These methods work. But they don't work how you think they do. What if we could help our bodies rebalance themselves instead of trying to cut corners with medication. Cutting corners in the long run convinces you that you know what you're doing, until you're challenged just a little too much.

When we take medication, it's like someone is reading for us instead of us learning how to read for ourselves. Sometimes we need someone to read for us, like when we're blind and our eyes don't work. The same goes for medication. Sometimes a part of our bodies cannot produce what they're meant to, like in the instance of insulin-dependent diabetes or menopause. In both instances, our bodies' tissues can't produce either insulin or estradiol. Sometimes the degree of damage on our bodies is so chronic or severe that they can't produce what's needed or even have the ability to function. In these cases, medication is often necessary and lifesaving. Even if we were to try and teach our bodies how to "read" by giving them all the resources, it doesn't matter. The organ is effectively blind.

But when our bodies' organs can function (see) just fine and they just haven't learned to read, if we continue to give medication to "read" for us, we never learn, and, in the long run, chronic disease occurs. Being able to see and having someone read for you only solves the surface issue. You never actually learn how to read, and you don't understand why you can't read. Is it that you don't know the alphabet? You can't spell? You can't string words together in a sentence? You're trying to read a completely different language and need a translator? When you dig deeper into the why, you'll unearth many reasons. The same is true for our bodies.

⁓

What I've found from my journey of continuing to ask why is that there are four main reasons why we have trouble "reading." I call these the 4 Female Fundamentals™.

Our bodies are made up of trillions of complex reactions, counterbalancing to each other every millisecond. These reactions are dependent on the balance of these four Fundamental levers.

1. Nervous system
2. Metabolism
3. Blood Sugars
4. Nutrients

Being finally relieved when someone can tell us what's going on is great and all, but it doesn't help explain why we have the issue. It's like someone saying, "You've got a really bland cake."

"No shit, sherlock. Are you going to tell me how and why?"

The same goes when someone tells you that you have endometriosis or migraines or IBS.

How you "fix" it is to first realize it's happening for a reason. It's a gift because it's showing you what you need to change in your external world or how you need to support your internal resources.

A DIAGNOSIS IS MUCH LIKE A CAKE

What type of cake you have depends on the ingredients you put into it. You can have all the right ingredients and get the ratios just right but if you put the oven on too hot, the cake will end up dry and burned. The same goes for if you have the oven set to the perfect temperature but your flour to milk ratio needs some improvement or, worse yet, you forgot to add the sugar. It's dependent on what raw materials (ingredients) your body has and the demands of the external environment (the oven temp).

If you have a terrible cake, you won't make a great cake until you understand why it was terrible in the first place.

So, if you've been diagnosed with something, know it's just telling you what type of cake you have. It's not telling you how you can change the recipe for a different result.

If I Wanted to Create a Recipe for Anxiety...

I'd have you believe that the anxiety was proof that you were broken. That there was something wrong with you. Add in an uncertain environment and give you no tools to know how to feel safe in your own body. Remove you from any social connections. Add some caffeine and a sugary breakfast, something like muesli and yogurt. Some iron deficiency and gut malabsorption. Create a salt imbalance in your brain. To top it off, I'd speed up your metabolism so your body felt like it needed to be ready to run or fight. Oh, and I'd take away physical exercise and sunlight.

If I Wanted to Create a Recipe for Mental Agility...

I'd have you believe that all emotions and experiences are valid. That they are designed to tell you something. Add in a calm environment and give you all the tools to self-regulate when the environment hasn't been so calm. Give you a small group of close, deep connections. I'd show you how to feel safe in your own body. I'd avoid caffeine first thing in the morning and have a high-protein and high-fat breakfast, something like eggs, meat, and veggies. Sprinkle in a happy gut that absorbs nutrients like a champion so your internal nutrients are nice and balanced. To top it off, I'd make your metabolism adaptive to whatever the demands are from the day and give it what it needs to return to a healthy baseline. Oh, and I'd lift weight (my own body weight or gym weights), get out in nature, and move my body in the sunshine.

The greatest myth we're told is that the "what" is the "why."

We become so swept up in what we "should" be doing that we forget that all we need to do is pay attention to what our bodies are telling us through our vast array of "big" and "small" symptoms. These messages give us the clues to how we need to support our body.

In the vast majority of cases, your body gets the perfect cake when you look after your 4 Female Fundamentals.

So, What Do I Actually Do?
The good news is that it's not that complicated
What I've learned from studying across multiple fields and continuously asking the question 'why?', is that ultimately our body is always looking out for us, always seeking balance. How it achieves this balance is through the 4 Fundamental functions

that all interconnect with each other. I call these the Female Fundamentals™ (They also benefit men too). When we look after the Female Fundamentals of our body, it's magic appears. We can stop looking for it externally, stop getting confused about what we need to do, the next health fad, bio hack or wonder drug, and become dialed into what our body is telling us it needs. That's all you need to do when you're lost in the space between.

Chapter 4

WELCOME TO THE
NEW WAY FORWARD...

~

The health and wellness industry is confusing as fuck.
When we focus on the Fundamentals, it becomes simple.

HELLO, FEMALE FUNDAMENTALS™

Do you feel like you're running around trying to find answers, a label, someone who can tell you what's going on with your body? You feel a mixture of confusion, frustration, hope, and this sense that you just want to know how (the fuck) to look after your body. It shouldn't be this complicated to be healthy, right? The health information out there isn't as "simple" as it once was—drink 2 liters of water, eat 5 pieces of vegetables, 3 pieces of fruit, some meat, throw some exercise and sleep in there too and you're set. Right?

Well, now we're told, you can't have this meat; you can't eat meat at all; only eat meat; you shouldn't eat between this time and that time; it's only about calories, but what about the nutrients—isn't food medicine? Only drink water from this place on a mountain, only do aerobic exercise; no, it's Pilates; no, it's HIIT workouts; HIIT is the devil; lift weights instead, but don't do it at the wrong time in your menstrual cycle. Oh, and don't forget to tape your mouth shut when you sleep, wake up with a freezing cold shower, and remember to breathe and be conscious about it… It's not surprising that we feel like we need a PhD to decipher something as simple as what the fuck we should eat for breakfast (or if you should skip it all together).

We have the right intentions. All we want is to give our bodies what they need to work at their best so we can go on living our lives. Our bodies are tools we use for life, not roadblocks. Looking after our bodies shouldn't feel like another full-time job, and it doesn't have to be. When we connect to our bodies and remember and trust that they know exactly what they're doing, we can wade through the sea of health and wellness advice with ease because we're using our bodies as a guide. We're focusing on the things that actually matter. We put the big rocks in before focusing on the little ones.

The things that actually matter are the 4 Female Fundamentals. Because they are what grounds and connects the human body with life. They are the four main levers the body uses to maintain balance and what sustains our lives, our survival.

> **"Get the fundamentals down and the level of everything you do will rise."**
> **— Michael Jordan**

THE FUNDAMENTALS DRIVING YOU

If we consider the 4 Female Fundamentals of our bodies like the needs of a car, it can be super simple to understand what our bodies need.

Nervous system = Driver

Metabolism = Structure and engine of the car

Nutrients = Fuel

Blood sugars = Mode of energy usage

1. Nervous System

Your car needs a driver. The driver is responsible for keeping the car safe by reacting to the demands of the external environment—the stop sign, the traffic lights, the other "crazy" or "calm" drivers on the road—and balancing that with the requirements inside the car (body)—distractions, the driver's stress, fatigue, alcohol intoxication, rushing and driving erratically, distractions from other passengers or, worse, from looking at their phone.

Your nervous system is your eyes, your ears; it's all of your senses taking in the internal and external information to tell your body how to respond to keep you safe and following the correct route. How it responds depends on its own state and the difficulty of the terrain. Who you allow to drive your car and have as passengers have a great impact on your ability to follow your GPS too. So, if you're feeling lost, confused, or out of control in your life, think about who you have given responsibility to for your health and life. Typically, the person we trust the most is often the person we give the responsibility of driving the car. If you're going on a family car trip, you wouldn't let the 9-year-old drive the car. *Giving yourself responsibility gives you more control.*

When your nervous system doesn't have what it needs, this knocks on to the other fundamentals. We fill up with the "wrong" fuel; we bump into things, rev the engine too high, and we forget to switch the mode of energy we're using.

2. Metabolism

Your car engine converts one form of energy into another. It converts chemical energy in the form of fuel into mechanical energy in the form of propulsion. In order for that to work efficiently, all of the structures of the car have to be functioning well. The engine, tires, spark plugs, radiator, car doors, the chassis. This is the same for your body.

Our cells are made up of these tiny components called organelles. They all have different vital functions that are necessary for metabolizing energy in our bodies, converting nutrients into life-sustaining energy. When these parts don't have what they need, our metabolism can speed up or slow down to try to compensate.

You need your metabolism to be functioning efficiently, much like a car with great fuel efficiency. When the car or cells start to become damaged, the efficiency is affected, creating a knock-on effect to the other Fundamentals.

3. Nutrients

Nutrients are the type of fuel you're putting into your car. You need to be consuming the type of fuel your body actually needs, but that's only just the beginning. The fuel needs to be absorbed and used alongside other nutrients in order to be utilized effectively—think fuel, oil, and radiator fluid—and toxins need to be excreted through your exhaust. When you're filling up your car with tainted fuel, or the fuel lines are leaky, or the exhaust is blocked, you'll run into trouble. The same is true in your body when it comes to nutrients.

Our nutrients facilitate communication between our cells. The exchange of our nutrients is how the body creates internal reactions. It's how nerve impulses are sent, how enzymes, hormones and proteins are made, and how our hearts contract. How our bodies know how much to sweat, to trigger an orgasm, to wake up feeling angry or energized. Nutrients are the fuel for every action in our body. The balance of nutrients is affected by the other Fundamentals.

4. Blood Sugars

The final thing to know about your body is that, much like in a hybrid car, it has developed two sources of energy so you will more than likely always have access to fuel for your car. This means that you always have a source of energy for your body. Even if you're without food in your fridge for a week, you can survive because you have stored energy.

In a hybrid car, we can use the fuel that we're pumping into the fuel lines from the tank, or we can use the stored fuel that's in the battery. The same is true for our bodies. We have access to our blood sugars for quick energy, and then we have our stored fuel in our liver and muscles, and fat for reserve energy. We need to have access to both sources at different times. When we do, our bodies can go further for longer. Blood sugars and our fuel "mode" impacts the other Fundamentals, and vice versa.

~~~

Most of the time, we jump into our cars and don't think twice about whether they're going to get us from A to B. We know they're going to facilitate our lives as we want them to. This is exactly like your body.

What happens if you're just starting out driving and your nervous system is a little worried because you don't have many skills? What if you're tired or if you're drunk? You would start to worry about whether the car would get you there. The same is true for your body.

What if you had a flat tire and have been driving around on the spare for a little longer than you know you should? This would make you question whether the car would get you to where you needed to go. The same is true for your body.

What if you filled up your tank at a dodgy looking petrol station, where the pump didn't work that well and you had a sneaking suspicion the fuel might be tainted? This would make you worried your car might not get you to where you want to go. The same is true for your body.

What if your hybrid isn't working so well, not clicking over to the reserve fuel as easily as it used to? This might make you worry that something was wrong with your car. The same is true for your body.

For our bodies to work, we need all parts of our "car" to be working. When one part isn't working too well, there are knock-on effects to the others.

EVERY FUNDAMENTAL REQUIRES CLOSE ATTENTION

**There isn't one Female Fundamental
that is more important than the other.**

Granted, there seems to be trends where different Fundamentals seem to be left to the last minute (*cough*, *cough*, nervous system), but even the zenniest of zen masters has to eat food, breathe, be in sunlight, and move their body. Just like it's not completely healthy to be someone who's outdoors, moving their body, and eating really well but is also stressed out of their mind… I'm sure we all know a few of those people. You might even be one of them.

I've met people who are hardworking farmers, who are outside, doing work that they love all day, eating foods that are grown from their farms, and have loving family and friends but are super stressed about how to make ends meet, what the weather is going to do, and how they can protect their livelihoods for years to come.

I've also met people who are successful business owners, who train for triathlons, eat only organic food, hell, even practically have their own wellness retreats at their houses with a sauna and ice bath, but everything is go-go-go. They develop chronic fatigue, iron deficiency, struggle with colds and flus for months, and even develop chronic conditions like autoimmune diseases.

We all know people on all sides of this. That's why looking after your health can seem so damn confusing.

~

One of my patients, Claire, used to think so too. She had been to naturopaths, doctors, tried various supplements and detoxes and still suffered from fatigue, debilitating period pain, skin and gut troubles. She was feeling defeated and thinking, *This must just be me. I just have to get used to this being normal.* She would find herself falling into patterns of beating herself up because she looked after herself well. She was in an amazing relationship with her supportive partner; she ate amazingly every day, hardly drank, and exercised most days.

So, what did Claire need to change? It seemed like everything was "perfect." When she came to me, I recommended we first do a hair tissue mineral analysis (HTMA). This is my favorite test when assessing functional health because it helps me objectively see how all four of the Female Fundamentals are functioning and gives a window (of up to three months) into the "why" behind her symptoms. Blood tests, on the other hand, are usually snapshots in time and are better at investigating for potentially life-threatening causes of illness.

Based on her results and her history, we found a clear pattern emerging in her Female Fundamentals. Her nervous system had been under such a high amount of stress for a long period of time that her body had decided the final thing it needed to do was slow down her metabolism to try and maintain balance. By slowing her metabolism, her thyroid and adrenal function had also decreased because they couldn't effectively keep up with the prolonged load. As a result of the slowed adrenals, thyroid, and metabolism, her ability to produce stomach acids and enzymes had decreased, contributing to her bloating as well as poor absorption of nutrients, even though she was eating well. Because she couldn't digest foods in the "right" area of her gut, this caused her to react to foods that are typically thought to be healthy, just because her body struggled to digest proteins, fats, and carbs in the part of the gut they were designed to be digested.

As a result of having a slowed metabolism and chronic stress, her body wanted to store energy (just in case) in the form of fat, and her nutrient ratios had altered to create these changes in her body. This contributed to bigger swings in moods around her periods, slowed gut motility and nutrient absorption, compromised excretion pathways, and poor thyroid and adrenal function. All of which contributed to the main concerns of her hormone imbalance, fatigue, and gut disturbance.

So, What Did We Do?

No, we didn't chase each symptom down a rabbit hole. We saw them as messages from the body telling us exactly what she needed.

Often, when we're in this state, it can be a challenge to make these changes because of the brain fog, the pain, the fatigue, the lack of trust in our bodies. It's tough to make changes when you don't have the raw materials in your body to be energized enough to make the changes in the first place.

So, we started Claire on a three-month course of specific supplements, based on her HTMA results, consisting of a combination of herbs and nutrients to help bring her metabolism back to a normal level, support her nervous system, boost gastric juices, and balance her nutrient requirements. But if we only changed her nutrients, we'd be band-aiding, because we needed to address all of her Fundamentals. So, we also made changes to her lifestyle using the 4 Female Fundamentals as a guide. She increased the variety of foods she consumed, reduced inflammatory foods, and implemented blood sugar hacks to minimize spikes from food across the day. She also understood the key factors triggering stress and actively adopted techniques to regulate her nervous system and reset her baseline.

The result... bowel movements multiple times a day, reduced period pain, clear head, and energy! Yay, Claire!

What Could Happen if You Don't Look After Your Female Fundamentals Over Time...

You might start out experiencing something like a trend I see among patients. You notice bloating, constipation, and diarrhea cycles, maybe some floating stools, brain fog, persistent fatigue, issues with your iron, and heavy periods. Often, a woman will notice these symptoms and visit her doctor or try to remedy each separate issue, like Jane who we met in Chapter 1. They're often told there's nothing wrong, or they're recommended medication to help with their symptoms without really understanding or being able to explain why it's happening in the first place. I see a lot of these women, and the overall feeling they have is frustration that no one can tell them why they feel how they do, and defeat because they feel like they have no other option other than to take the treatment for something they don't even know is causing their symptoms.

What we know is that these symptoms are not separate issues. Remember, we're one system made up of many parts, not many separate systems. When we view our bodies in silos (addressing "parts" in isolation), we can give ourselves momentary relief, much like fast food. However, if we fast-forward five years, a typical patient, under the self-guidance of addressing separate symptoms, will need their gallbladder removed. Further into the future, she can develop heavier periods, some uterine fibroids and need a hysterectomy. Then, eventually, she'll be placed on thyroid medication because her metabolism will have significantly slowed. She'll probably suffer from osteoporosis and cardiovascular disease in her later years of life. This is a common physiological trend seen among female patients.

What Happens When we Know Our Bodies are the Solution?

What if she looks at the bloating, constipation, heavy and painful periods, fatigue, and changes to hair not as a sign that there is something wrong with her, but as a gift from the body telling her what she needs to change?

We don't need to know how each different pathway in the body interrelates; all we need to know is that when all four of the Female Fundamentals have what they need, we can balance our internal resources with the demands of the external world. When this happens, our symptoms fall away because we're not surviving—we're thriving.

～～

Same patient, different perspective…

The hair loss, fatigue, constipation, and bloating are all signs that the body is slowing down. It could be perceived that the stress she feels is best handled by freezing, or fawning, so her metabolism is slowed initially. We see this in animals when they "play dead." Their heart rates slow, blood pressure lowers, and all bodily functions slow down to conserve energy for survival.

For this to happen, her body will slow the thyroid gland. When this occurs, her parathyroid gland function increases in a bid to maintain balance. The parathyroid gland is largely responsible for knowing where to put the calcium in our bodies. Is it going to store it in our bones? Or is it going to pull more into the bloodstream? Kind of like having money stored in the bank or ready for use in your wallet. When our thyroid slows down, due to either initial freeze/fawn response or prolonged fight-or-flight response, our parathyroid glands increase activity, leading to a need for more calcium in the blood.[17] They're doing this to help us cope with the level of stress our bodies perceive.

When calcium is higher in the blood, combined with slowed gut motility and underfunctioning thyroid, emptying of the gallbladder slows, creating calcium deposits in the organ. These deposits form gallstones. When we fix this issue by removing the gallbladder, the stones are removed, but the reason why the stones are there in the first place continues. Over time, the higher amounts of calcium in the blood can lead to uterine fibroids—commonly seen with heavy menstrual cycles in later life—breakthrough bleeding, and a feeling of fullness in the lower abdomen. Depending on the stage of life you're in, where the fibroids are, and the severity of your symptoms, you may be offered hysterectomy or a myomectomy to "fix" the problem, but the underlying pattern of an underfunctioning thyroid and overfunctioning parathyroid gland continues.

Finally, you reach a point where your blood tests are bad enough to warrant thyroid medication. Which typically only helps to support the inactive thyroid hormone (T4) and doesn't help with the conversion of the inactive form to the active form (T3) that your body uses. This conversion is dependent on stress levels, nutrient levels, and absorption and excretion processes in the body. So you can end up on a lifetime of thyroid medication. The underlying mechanism still continues, and your bones are leaching nutrients into the bloodstream, you've been diagnosed with osteopenia or osteoporosis and told to start taking vitamin D, calcium and vitamin K2. These nutrients are meant to help boost the amount of calcium in the bones. But when the master controller of where calcium sits in the body is telling your body it needs to be in circulation not in storage (bone), then this pattern can continue. Leading to higher likelihood of cardiovascular disease.

See how everything is linked?

NERVOUS SYSTEM
The driver of your car.

Your driver decides where you're going. Their job is to read the external environment and make sure they can adapt and stay safe. Watch out for kangaroos, read traffic lights, know how to merge, and read traffic. Their job is to also make sure the inside car environment is ideal. Have you ever tried to drive with a car full of drunk people screaming? Or a car full of kids excited for a 5-year-old's birthday party? It's difficult to focus and stay safe when your internal environment is chaotic.

Many factors can affect how well your nervous system drives, for example: You could lack proper guidance and the raw skills to know how to drive. This can happen when we're brought up in environments that are emotionally volatile, where we're not shown or given skills to regulate our nervous systems. Other times, it can be a raw material that we're lacking in our internal environments that make it difficult to adapt, much like trying to drive blindfolded. Lacking appropriate nutrients to make neurotransmitters and riding sugar roller-coasters can leave you feeling anxious, even though you might be still, like a parked car.

The driver's job is to follow the GPS by adapting and making sure the internal car environment and external road environment are safe. When the nervous system is out of whack, we can stop paying attention to the GPS and not realize we've gone offtrack. Or when we do realize we've gone offtrack, it becomes a big deal. Think about when you're running late for something and you go the wrong way. This can further agitate your nervous system.

The Truth About Stress

What we deem stress is a response to those environments. Stress causes us to adapt. When we have resources to adapt to the stress and return to baseline, the stress creates positive adaptations in our bodies. Like when a baby learns to roll, to sit, to crawl, and to walk. Stress is involved in the learning process.

When we don't have the resources to adapt to the stress, or if we find it difficult to return to baseline and, as a result, stay in stress, the adaptation starts to become negative. Like when you're studying for exams or going through a divorce and your health falls in a heap once it's done.

Stress comes in all different shapes and sizes. At its core, it's a challenge for the body, and challenges can be perceived as either good or bad. How we perceive stress determines whether it affects us negatively, for example, causing health issues and premature death, or positively, creating evolution and adaptation within the body.

One surprising study found that stress alone isn't a killer; it's the belief that stress is harmful to our health that can send us packing early.[18] That's right. People previously thought to be dying prematurely from stress were actually dying from the belief that stress would kill them, a self-fulfilling prophecy. So, when it comes to stress, it's worth paying attention to your perception— more on this in chapter 5.

What Exactly is the Nervous System?

Broadly speaking, the nervous system is split into the automatic and nonautomatic parts: the autonomic and somatic.

The automatic part of the nervous system is responsible for the trillions of reactions happening right this second to keep you alive, balancing your body temperature, making your heart beat, creating energy, hormones, brain impulses, gastric juices, and sweat responses, dilating your pupils, and keeping a keen eye on the smells around you.

We can think of how it works like a traffic light. It's split up into three main functions. Green lights, orange lights, and red lights. Researcher Dr. Stephen Porges termed this "polyvagal theory."[19] Just like a traffic light, neither the green, orange, or red light is bad. Sure, we all want green lights, but imagine if we actually had nothing but green lights. There would be accidents happening everywhere. There would be no order. We need to be able to have all three levels. The trouble comes when we're always going, always stopping, or always just making it.

Green Lights

This is where we want to exist most of the time. It feels like an ease and flow. We often feel a sense of pleasure, play, and curiosity. Think about when you're going for a drive and every set of lights you hit is green. It feels amazing, and the drive goes smoothly. You often arrive at your destination feeling calm.

When we're in the green, this is what's called our ventral vagal mode.

When you're in this mode, you can feel

- Safe
- Grounded
- Curious
- Playful
- Pleasure
- Compassionate

- Grateful
- Present
- Connected
- Calm
- Creative

It's no surprise that when we drive through green lights more often, we feel more like "ourselves."

Behaviors often look like

- Responding instead of reacting
- Experiencing more curiosity as opposed to judgment
- Ability to connect and relate to others
- Prosperity and vitality in the voice
- Posture is automatically more upright and open
- Creativity flows
- Slower walking and talking
- Playful energy
- Waking up energized
- A sense of hope
- Excitement

Thoughts often sound like

- I feel safe.
- Everything is working out for me.
- I have so much love for this person.
- That is wonderful.
- This food that I'm eating tastes delicious!

- I love life.
- I have so much love for myself.
- I wonder... (you've got time to daydream).
- I'm exactly where I need to be.
- Mmmmmmhhh.

So, what's happening inside your body?

- What functions improve?
    - ~ Digestion and intestinal motility
    - ~ Rest
    - ~ Health and vitality
    - ~ Oxytocin (pleasure hormone)
    - ~ Resistance to infections
    - ~ Blood supply to non-vital organs (like skin and extremities)
    - ~ Heart rate variability (a sign that your nervous system is adaptable)

- What decreases?
    - ~ Defensive responses

Our bodies choose the green light mode, the ventral vagal response, when it's the response they perceive they need. If we want to be in this mode more often, we can alter our environments and support our internal nutrients to find this balance.

Ideally, for longevity and overall health, we want to be able to return to this baseline of green lights frequently. However, always getting green lights is dangerous because we won't have any protective mechanisms for survival.

Orange Lights

Orange lights are our sympathetic mode, our fight-or-flight.

They feel like a rush and a buildup of tension. Think about when you've gone for a drive and every time you go through a set of lights, it's orange. What happens? You grip the wheel a little tighter; your hands are sweaty. Your foot gets a little tense wondering whether it needs to stay on the accelerator or quickly jump to the brake; your eyes widen and dart from left to right to make sure other cars aren't coming; your breath becomes a little shallower; your heart rate quickens, and your bum cheeks might even tighten too.

When you're in this mode, you can feel

- Panic
- Fear
- Anxiety
- Rage
- Anger
- Irritation
- Worry or concern
- Frustration

Behaviors often look like

- Avoiding replying back to messages
- Ghosting people
- Defensiveness in arguments

- Quick to judge other people and make them wrong
- Feeling like you're in a rush and don't have enough time
- Tailgating people in your car
- Binge eating when you realize you forgot to eat breakfast or lunch
- Walking fast
- Talking fast
- Sensitive to light and needing a dark room to sleep
- Needing sunglasses outside all the time
- Tight hamstrings and chest
- Picking fights
- Sensitive to sound and needing to sleep with earplugs in, or waking up to small sounds throughout the night

Thoughts often sound like

- I don't have time for this.
- Can everyone get off my back?
- Everyone is looking at me.
- Why is everyone attacking me?
- If I just quickly do this, then…
- I wish I could clone myself, then I could get everything done.
- I have 20 minutes for morning meditation, then I need to get 50 things on my to-do list done.

What's happening in your body?

- What increases?
    - ~ Heart rate.

- ~ Blood pressure.
- ~ Blood sugar—your body wants more energy ready, so it brings it into the blood.
- ~ Pupil size.
- ~ Adrenaline.
- ~ Cortisol.
- ~ Blood clotting—because your body is thinking you're under threat and may be attacked and bleed out.
- ~ Sweating.

- What decreases?
  - ~ Fuel storage—because you want quick access to fuel.
  - ~ Digestion—it's not important when you're under threat. Stomach acid production can increase initially; pancreatic enzymes decrease.
  - ~ Heart rate variability.
  - ~ Salivation—ever get a dry mouth before you've had to give a speech? This is why.
  - ~ Immune response—ever notice how you get sick after a big, stressful event, like exams, business events, or a wedding?
  - ~ Blood supply to extremities—hello, cold hands and feet, which are also probably a little sweaty.

Conditions associated with prolonged sympathetic activation (orange lights)[20]

- Anxiety
- Multiple sclerosis
- Bacterial infections
- Hyperthyroidism
- Hodgkin's disease
- Ulcers (stomach and duodenal)
- Allergies
- Rheumatoid arthritis

Red Lights

Red lights are also known as our dorsal vagal nervous system. We have two main types of behaviors here: freezing and fawning.

Freezing is like when you're stopped at a red light and you completely zone out, disassociate, and don't realize the light has turned green until you get a toot from behind.

You can think of fawning as turning your blasting music down at the red traffic light to not draw too much attention to yourself. It's all about adapting and pleasing others to maintain your safety.

When you're in this mode, you can feel

- Numb
- Trapped
- Hopeless
- Disassociated
- Depressed
- Helpless
- High pain threshold

Behaviors can look like

- Putting others' needs before your own
- Apologizing and saying sorry all the time
- Forgetting to eat breakfast or lunch
- Forgetting what you're doing halfway through doing it
- Living from other people's perspectives
- Occasional slow, deep breathing
- High pain threshold

Fawn

- People-pleasing
- Codependency
- Lack of boundaries

Freeze

- Disassociation
- Numbness
- Shutting down
- Low energy

Thoughts can often sound like

- I better not ask for help because that will inconvenience someone else.
- I'm a burden.
- If I do X, Y, Z, they will be happy.
- I wonder what that person thinks of me.
- Why can't my body keep up with me?

- I'm usually really good at coping, why is my body being affected now?

What's happening in your body?

Like the fancy cars that automatically turn off when you stop at a traffic light, the body wants and needs rest and refueling.

- What increases?
  - ~ Fuel storage and insulin activity—your body wants to store your energy as fat, as this is seen as best for survival. Typically, this fat is stored around the abdomen, hips, and thighs.
  - ~ Pain-numbing endorphins.
  - ~ Thirst, salt cravings, urination, and water retention due to low salt (particularly sodium and potassium).

- What decreases?
  - ~ Basal body temperature
  - ~ Basal metabolic rate
  - ~ Heart rate
  - ~ Heart rate variability
  - ~ Blood pressure
  - ~ Facial expressions and eye contact
  - ~ Sexual responses, expression, and ability to become aroused and orgasm
  - ~ Immune response

Conditions associated with prolonged dorsal parasympathetic activation (red lights)[21]

- Osteoarthritis
- PMS
- Lupus
- Anorexia[22]
- Adult-onset diabetes
- Hypothyroidism
- Stomach ulcers
- Viral infections

~

Like with the flags in the last chapter, you can be colorblind to the lights too. You can convince yourself that a red light is actually a green light, running red light after red light after red light, trying to keep going when your body is screaming at you to stop. Stopping isn't a bad thing. Stopping allows for the flow of traffic. Even your car runs out of fuel and must stop to refuel at some point. When you continue to run red lights in your car, you get pulled over by the police. When you do it in your body, you get picked up by an ambulance.

How Do You Know if You're Running Red Lights?

You're waking up tired, going to bed tired, and being fueled by a to-do list. If you could wave a magic fairy wand and say that everything was done—no washing to do, no one to see, no work to do, nowhere to go—what would you do? If your answer is "sleep" or "nothing," you're running red lights, and your to-do list is making you color-blind.

The thing to remember about each response of your autonomic nervous system is that it is healthy. Just like we need to have green, orange, and red lights for the roads to be safe, all parts of our nervous system are vital for our survival. There's no use having green lights every time we all reach an intersection. Can you imagine the carnage? In the same way, it's dangerous to have our bodies feel "safe" all the time. If that were reality, the human race would have died off a long time ago. The body's unique design keeps us alive and helps us adapt to our environments to become even stronger and evolve as a species. The issue comes when we stay in one zone for too long and the response isn't as adaptable as it once was. You get sick and instead of taking a week to get over it, you're sick for months on end. You develop autoimmune issues, hormonal imbalances, IBS, fertility struggles, migraines, acne, PCOS, endometriosis, thyroid issues. Why? Because of the knock-on effects that can be happening to your other Female Fundamentals.

If you get stressed over having everything perfect for your health, the stress could kill you faster than the perfection is supposedly healing you.

What Changes the Color of the Lights?

Different levels of stress lead to the nervous system changing light colors.

Stress can come in many different forms:

> ~ **Chemical:** Infections, active disease process, inflammation, heavy metals, lack of nourishment
>
> ~ **Physical:** Physical trauma, exercise, body posture
>
> ~ **Emotional:** Varied different emotional states

The degree to which your body perceives it can cope with this stress determines what light it chooses to be in. It's why when you have an infection, you develop a fever—your body goes into an orange light. When you suddenly hurt yourself without warning and you feel like you're going to pass out, your body goes into a red light. When you go to a market and feel calm and peaceful, while your friend feels panicked, your body has chosen a green light, and your friend's has chosen the orange light. All of these responses are exactly what the body perceives it needs to do to ensure your survival and maintain balance.[23]

Signs Your Nervous System Needs Support:

- You get headaches towards the end of the day.
- Your pupils are always large.
- You have trouble with getting to sleep or staying asleep (waking up every 2–3 hours).
- Hair loss.
- Persistent gut issues, food intolerances.
- Feel simultaneously tired and wired.
- If you didn't have a to-do list or have a resistance to being seen as lazy, you would happily be in bed all day.

- Poor posture.
- Tight hips.
- Baseline anxiety or depression.
- Low tolerance to stress.
- Inability to sit still or in "boredom."
- Poor sleep.

You Don't Know What You Don't Know

When I was in my early 20s, like many people, I started working full-time. After a few months, I started to develop this feeling of heaviness in both of my legs. There was nothing physically happening with my spine, pelvis, or nerves, so I went to the doctor to get some blood tests done. I thought maybe I had iron deficiency, even though I had never struggled with this before. She ran a whole host of tests looking for infections and checking iron, thyroid, blood sugars, kidney and liver function. All of them came back normal. She then asked me what had been going on in my life. After I had explained the last six months of my life, she said, "Do you think there is a chance you could be stressed?" At the time, I truly didn't think I was under that much stress compared to moments in the past. Looking back now, my body *was* stressed.

I see this in patients frequently. Often, they're so adapted to their prolonged state of stress that it feels "normal." But when we see the results of their functional tests, health, history, and demeanor their body is saying otherwise.

The Golden Rules for Supporting the Nervous System

The best place for our bodies to be the majority of the time is in "green lights." Being able to recalibrate and return to green lights without getting stuck in your orange (sympathetic) or red (dorsal vagal) lights is critical for supporting your nervous system. There are several ways you can achieve this:

- **Connect to your body:** This helps you make decisions from your body and use your mind as a resource. Make time for yourself. Be a savage at putting yourself first.

- **Connect with others:** We need others for survival. If you can connect to yourself first, it will help determine who you want around you and who you don't.

- **Use pace to change your state:** When you feel like you're in a rush, walk and talk half a second slower. If you feel like you're in a slump, put on some music and jump or dance around.

- **Watch your posture:** When our shoulders slump forward and round, this activates what are called our second order sympathetic neurons in the middle of our backs, causing the body to think it's under threat, sending it into "orange light" territory.[24] The famous Amy Cuddy Ted Talk speaks to how standing in a "superhero pose" can change your internal hormones and leave you feeling more certain, creative, and connected—that is, green lights.

- **Singing**: This activates the part of your brain that wakes up when in "green lights."

- **Mind the light:** Too much artificial light can trigger your orange lights.
- **Breath**: Rapid breathing triggers orange lights; slowed breathing triggers red lights, and controlled and focused breathing helps bring you into green lights.
- **Movement**: Movements help our brains in many ways, including stimulating the cerebellum, which acts like a battery for the upper cortex. As I am initially trained as a chiropractor, I know that restoring movement to all of the joints and muscles of the body, so that it acts symmetrically, is also high on the list of helping the body and brain to better coordinate. When the brain's higher cortex is stimulated through better body movement, it reduces the length of time we're in orange and red lights by helping the responsive part of our brains become more stimulated than our reactive brains. In short, move to move into green lights.

What Can You Do to Support Your Nervous System?

You can support your nervous system by doing things your body wouldn't normally do if it were under attack, such as:

- Walking half a second slower
- Talking half a second slower
- Dancing naked in the kitchen or bedroom
- Skipping
- Art and other creative projects
- Lying on the ground with your legs and arms stretched out like a starfish

Get creative and find things that bring you a sense of joy, pleasure, creativity, or play.

The main goal is to be going through green lights most of the time and to be able to progress through each of the different zones without getting stuck for too long (our environments can cause our bodies to be stuck in those states).

Remember… *Your body is always having a healthy response to an abnormal environment.*

That environment can be internal, in terms of our raw materials, or external. A cornerstone for being able to go to green lights is safety. Safety in our bodies and safety in our environments. We can establish safety in our bodies when we learn to trust ourselves and our bodies, and live in a safe environment. If you feel like you're in an unsafe environment, no amount of "health hacks" will outweigh this, and you should seek whatever assistance needed to get yourself into a safer situation.

Quiz on Nervous System

If you want to find out what nervous system state you're in, take the free Female Fundamentals quiz on our website: www.femalefundamentals.com.au/resources.

METABOLISM
Structure and engine.

Metabolism is just like the engine and structure of your car. It turns fuel into motion. The more the engine works, the hotter

it gets. The same is true for your body. The faster your metabolism gets, the hotter you become—body temperature, that is.
Hotter and faster doesn't necessarily mean better though. Cars
can overheat.

Much like a car needs pumped-up tires, spark plugs, an alter-
nator, radiator, pistons (yes, pistons sound important) to be able to
use fuel and turn it into movement, our bodies' needs must also
be met in order to move well. Complex reactions take place inside
our cells, which contain many different parts, just like a car engine,
except they have names like mitochondria, cytoplasm, ribosomes,
and smooth endoplasmic reticulum. The good news is you don't
have to remember any of those things, like how you don't need to
know how to fix your own car; you just need to know when to take
it to the mechanic and how to best look after it.

How Do You Know When Your Metabolism Needs Support?

Let's clear up the elephant in the room. We often think of metabolism as how well our bodies can handle eating crappy foods.
The common thinking is that if you can eat crap food, or a lot of
food, and not gain weight, then you're "one of the lucky ones"
with a fast metabolism. On the other hand, if you eat practically
nothing and do gain weight, you're "unlucky" and stuck with a
slow metabolism.

I used to think like this too. What I've found after working with
hundreds of patients is that patients who could "eat anything and
stay skinny" could often have slow metabolisms, and those who

would restrict calories and exercise every day could often have fast metabolisms. Still not convinced? Think of a friend you know who eats terribly and doesn't exercise, yet they're skinny. Conversely, we know people who have immaculate diets and exercise almost every day, yet they can't seem to lose weight. The fallacy is that we convince ourselves that they're "lazy." We can drop that belief at the door. Weight and metabolism are correlated, but they aren't inextricably linked.

The good news is metabolism, like whether your engine is working well or not, isn't luck, since weight has many other variables, including the balance of hormones: insulin, thyroxine, melatonin, ghrelin, and leptin. It's not purely a metabolism issue.

How Does Our Metabolism Work?

Our metabolism is largely connected to an "engine part" called the mitochondria. How fast or slow the mitochondria and metabolism function is dependent on the movement of nutrients throughout the cell, largely phosphorus and calcium.

This is important because it ties into our other Fundamentals.

When the nervous system is in an orange light state, it wants to speed up. It's in fight-or-flight, so it dumps calcium. Because calcium is a sedative to cells, it slows them down, which may seem counterintuitive when the nervous system wants us to speed up. When it does this, our metabolic rate speeds up, which is often why we feel hot and flustered when we're stressed. Our metabolic rate, much like an engine, has been driving fast, causing the engine to get hot.

When the nervous system has been in an orange light for a long period, it eventually turns red because we've depleted a lot of our stimulatory nutrients, just like when we keep driving through orange lights and finally decide to stop at the next one. When we're at a red light (freeze/fawn) response, our body wants to retain calcium because it slows us down. It deems this necessary for trying to maintain balance. We all need rest and if we don't take it and continue to go through orange lights, our body will force us into a red light by retaining calcium.

When there's less calcium in our tissues, our body can have trouble releasing insulin from the pancreas, leading to higher blood sugars—perfect for an orange light state. When our metabolism slows due to our body retaining more calcium and wanting to rest at a red light, we can experience lower blood sugars.

What this looks like...

Have you ever known someone to experience acute stress and lose weight initially? Their body went into an orange light, and their metabolism sped up. If that stress hangs around for a long period of time, the person often ends up gaining weight. Why? Because their metabolism changed over time, resulting in the nervous system altering nutrients, blood sugars and the balance of the metabolism.

Does this mean you should change how much calcium you consume?

Not entirely. Remember, your body is like a mum who feeds her kids snacks. She needs to keep track of how many snacks she has in reserve for emergencies and how much she has given to the toddler. So, where your calcium is in your body, whether it's in reserve or in the bloodstream, is dependent on the demand of the toddler and the number of snacks you have.

When the toddler wants to run around and have a lot of energy, they don't need many snacks. Our bodies don't give them much calcium because that would slow the toddler down. It's the last thing they want.

When the toddler has run around and is now exhausted and starting to teeter on the side of a tantrum, Mum saves the day by giving them a snack, boosting calcium levels to calm them and slow them down.

We still need to be consuming calcium (buying snacks), but how they're divided up and when they're given is dependent on the perceived needs of the toddler—that is, your body's relationship with its environment. Balance. It's all about balance.

The calcium balance is determined by what you're consuming and what your body needs.

What Determines if You're a Slow or Fast Metabolizer?

Contrary to what you might believe, your metabolism can be changed. How your metabolism functions is dependent on multiple factors.

Environmental factors that aren't so easily changed, like inheriting your parents' mineral profiles, the eating patterns of your family, and living in similar environments to your family, can contribute to genetic similarities. It has been found that children with the same mineral patterns as their parents are predisposed to similar health conditions as well as personality traits. Does anxiety run in your family, or does it run in your mineral patterns?

Other factors, which are more readily changed, are things like starvation, stress, and sickness.

A fast or a slow metabolic rate isn't better or worse than the other. The key is being able to adapt, just like a car. We don't want to be stuck driving 20 km/h, just like we don't want to be stuck driving 100 km/h. Ideally, we want a metabolism that has what it needs to adapt its speed as the environment changes. Like everything in the body, the metabolism isn't stagnant. Whether it's fast or slow is dependent on how it perceives it needs to respond to the environment to keep you alive.

WHAT METABOLIC TYPE ARE YOU?

Slow Metabolism

The body of a slow metabolizer is like a car stuck driving 20 km/h on a highway. They often want to go and go and go, but their body is struggling to keep up with them.

Slow metabolizers want to hold on to more sedative nutrients so the body can heal. To do this, the body's parathyroid function and pancreatic function increase, and the thyroid and adrenals become sluggish. This creates a slowed metabolic rate because the body holds on to more sedative minerals like calcium and magnesium. You can think of it like giving your toddler snacks that make them sleepy. An example of this is how nutrients in breast milk soothe babies and why magnesium is given to relax muscles.

Signs of a slowed metabolism

- Tendency to gain weight in the abdomen, hips, and thighs.
- Dizzy when standing too quickly—adrenals aren't working quick enough to alter blood pressure with the demands of gravity, resulting in a woozy feeling.
- Poor circulation.
- Cold hands and feet.
- Waking up frequently throughout the night.
- Increased levels of insulin, which may contribute to hypoglycemia.
- Slow hair and nail growth.
- Dry skin.

Things that slow your metabolic rate

- Significant illness
- Chronic stress
- High dietary fat intake
- Poor sleep
- Heavy metals and environmental toxins
- Significant, prolonged calorie restriction

- Blue light
- Heat exposure
- EMFs (electromagnetic fields)[25]

Fast Metabolism

The body of a fast metabolizer is like a car stuck driving 100 km/h in a 40 km/h zone. Their body is often moving fast and has difficulty slowing down. We often think being a fast metabolizer is a good thing; however, when your car doesn't have enough resources, like coolant and oil, racing it around the block isn't the smartest move. It can result in the engine overheating and the car being forced to slow down. There's a reason why it's called *burnout.* It's not about fast or slow; it's about having enough nutrients to be capable of either speed.

Our metabolism increases because we have more stimulatory nutrients than we do sedative nutrients. Just like when you've accidentally given your toddler a snack full of sugar and salt, they're going to be bouncing off the walls.

Signs of a fast metabolism

- Increased sweating
- Difficulty sitting still
- Decreased levels of insulin, contributing to hyperglycemia
- Weight gain around the arms, back, and abdomen
- Hot body temperature
- Easily agitated
- Tend to gravitate towards chaotic environments

- Addictive type personalities
- Often addicted to stress, caffeine, and stimulation

Things that quicken your metabolic rate

- Acute stress
- Acute illness
- Ovulation
- Cold exposure
- Sunlight (UVA)
- Protein

Foods Impact Your Metabolism

Often, when we're trying to lose weight, we first alter the ratio between our protein, fat, and carbohydrates, or completely cut out one of them all together—in the case of keto, largely removing carbohydrates. The food and diet industry loves to demonize and glamourize different macronutrients from time to time.

What you need to remember is that all foods increase our metabolic rate to some degree. Protein increases our metabolic rate the most, followed by carbohydrates, and, finally, fats. When we understand our baseline metabolic type, we can use this knowledge to our advantage. If our current metabolic rate is slow, we can help to increase it by consuming more protein. However, if our metabolic rate is already fast, increasing protein can contribute to creating an even further imbalance. Instead, we should aim to have an equal balance between proteins, fats, and carbs.

Your Food Cravings are Your Body Talking to You...

We crave high-fat foods like chocolate before our periods because they have a sedative and calming effect on our bodies. This helps regulate our moods because the natural fall in progesterone just before our periods can reduce our stress resilience. The same goes for milk and cheese—they're high-fat foods that can help by calming the nervous system. Craving a greasy, fatty meal for a hangover? Well, there's a reason for it. Alcohol increases anxiety networks in the brain, and fatty food helps regulate our moods.

How to Support Your Metabolism?

Balance your other Female Fundamentals

Our metabolism is always altering to try and find balance with our nervous system, nutrients, and blood sugars. If we want to alter our metabolism, we first need to look at the messages our other fundamentals are sending. Is our nervous system in an orange or red light? Do we have enough nutrients to sustain the demands of our lives? What are our blood sugars doing? The best way to care for our metabolism is to give our car engines everything they need.

Light, sunlight, and EMFs

The sun is like the ignition that turns our engines on. No ignition, no start to the metabolism. This is why we often see weight gain occur when our sleep and circadian rhythms have been changed, and in the darker winter months.[26]

In addition to the ignition, we also need our cars to be full of nutrients (fuel) for the ignition to start the engine. This is why not only our macronutrient but also our micronutrient balance is important.

To support your metabolism with sunlight, expose yourself to the sun as close to sunrise and sunset as you can. This helps your body receive "UVA" light, a wavelength of sunlight that helps your cells generate energy.[27]

All light isn't created equal... For example, blue light like that from TV, computer, and phone screens, and electromagnetic fields (EMFs) from technological devices can contribute to leptin resistance. Leptin is a hormone that tells our bodies the levels of our fat stores. When we become resistant to this, we can feel hungry and consume more food even when we have high levels of fat storage. The increased amount of fat contributes to higher insulin levels and a slowed metabolic rate, which makes it more difficult to lose weight, creating a vicious cycle. Minimizing blue light and exposure to EMFs helps our bodies become more leptin sensitive, making it easier to break the cycle.[28]

Earthing

A by-product of our metabolism is energy. Our mitochondria produce this energy by swapping negative and positive charge. It's important for our mitochondria to maintain this balance of positive and negative charge for energy to be produced and dispersed. Just like a battery has a positive and negative charge and a magnet has a positive and negative pole, so do our cells.

Some of the best ways to maintain this balance are walking in nature barefoot and inhaling air from the fresh ocean, around a waterfall, or in a rainforest. This is because the earth's surface and the air are full of negative ions, which balance out the positive charge that occurs in our bodies from producing energy. It's like clearing out the exhaust of each of our cells, removing toxins and damaged cells as well as improving our metabolism.

Expose yourself to cold and heat

Just as our breath changes with the state of stress we're in—orange light, it quickens; red light, it slows—the body's temperature changes depending on the speed of the metabolism. When we remember that our bodies are always capable of change and their number one job is to achieve balance with the external environment, we can adapt how they behave by changing our environments.

Doing this in a way that challenges our bodies just enough can generate a healthy and beneficial level of stress. Since the metabolism changes body temperature, if we want to change our metabolism from the outside in, we can do so by altering the external temperature.

This is why cold ice baths and saunas can be effective, triggering chemicals called heat shock and cold shock proteins. In ice baths, the cellular metabolism wants to speed up to keep us warm. In saunas, it wants to slow us down to avoid overheating. When we remember this, we can more adequately support our bodies.

If you're a fast type, you'll often find saunas relaxing because they help to balance your metabolism. If you're a slow type, *after* an ice bath, you'll often feel invigorated as your metabolism speeds up in an effort to regulate balance. Remember to first check that your cardiovascular system isn't already under extreme stress before attempting ice baths or sauna treatment. Get your blood pressure and heart function checked prior to starting, and remember, it's one step at a time. Pay attention to how your body feels and use it, not your Instagram algorithm, as a guide.

Quiz on Metabolism

If you want to find out what metabolic type you are, take the free Female Fundamentals quiz on our website: www.femalefundamentals.com.au/resources.

NUTRIENTS
Fuel.

Our nutrients are like the fuel we give to our cars. Have you accidentally filled up your diesel car with unleaded petrol? Generally, it doesn't end well. Along with filling up our cars with the correct fuel, we also must be able to get the fuel to the engine, absorbing nutrients and getting rid of by-products through the exhaust. You can be using the highest-quality, premium food, or fuel, but if your body, or car, can't absorb or excrete it, you'll start to run into trouble.

Nutrients are as simple as:

1. What am I consuming or exposing myself to (that is, what's coming in)?
2. Can I absorb and use these nutrients?
3. Am I able to get rid of the waste products?

Let's discuss each point in more detail.

WHAT ARE YOU CONSUMING OR EXPOSING YOURSELF TO?

Diets, what we put in our mouths, on our skin, and into our environments are possibly the most hotly debated topics in the healthcare industry, and, for many people, they create a lot of mental load throughout the day.

Don't eat meat; only eat meat; fish is good for you; fish is full of mercury; fat is the devil; add fat to your coffee; don't drink coffee; only get food on the outside lanes of the supermarket; supermarket fruit is nutrient-depleted and covered in toxic sprays; we need supplements because our food isn't as nutrient-dense as it once was; supplements are a waste of money—you just wee them out; sugar-free is good for you; sugar free means it's full of chemicals; aspartame is cancer-causing; big companies are just making up research results to sell products; if the label has a number on it, don't eat it; don't even get me started on gluten; don't drink milk (but cheese and chocolate are fine); don't touch anything stored in plastic; only eat organic; organic is just a fake label that lets them charge more; avoid

FODMAP foods; food is medicine; it doesn't matter what you eat, just balance the calories… what about fiber? We can't forget fiber. Was I meant to eat more fiber or less? Oh, and the microbiome.

I'm getting whiplash just reading this. On any given day, we can go on our social media feeds and find all of this information. In fact, at any given moment, you could find any of this by doing a Google search or even a search of research databases.

~

We can convince ourselves of anything, particularly when we're looking for answers outside of ourselves, the ones that fit the narrative we want. It's called confirmation bias, and it's where marketing comes in. When we've been persuaded to think of our bodies as inherently broken, complicated, or fragile, we can get caught up in the confusion of looking for answers in external sources (I know I've mentioned this about 500 times already, but I really want it to sink in—it's about time we heard a new narrative!).

So, how do we make it simple? Think about what your body and cells need because, really, your body is a meat suit made up of around 32 trillion cells. How these cells work is largely dependent on their exchange of different nutrients.

We need a mixture of macro and micronutrients for our bodies to create things like enzymes, hormones, muscle contractions, emotions of anxiety, anger, love, for our nerve impulses to move our limbs to hug a loved one, for our eyes to see and our skin to glow.

All food groups are important.

Macronutrients

Protein

Protein breaks down into smaller molecules called amino acids. Both proteins and amino acids are the building blocks for hormones such as thyroxine, adrenaline, dopamine, melatonin, serotonin, oxytocin, prolactin, GnRH, and insulin. They help to stabilize mood, regulate the sleep wake cycle, boost energy and libido as well as ovulation.

Fat

Fat is essential for the production of lipid-based hormones such as cholesterol, cortisol, progesterone, estrogen, androgens, and aldosterone. It also allows us to utilize fat-soluble vitamins like vitamin A, D, E, and K. These hormones and vitamins are essential to the menstrual cycle, wound healing, stress response, libido, ovulation, immune system, bone health, hair growth and loss as well as detoxification.

Carbohydrates

Carbohydrates combine with proteins to form what are called glycoproteins. They create hormones such as follicle stimulating hormone (FSH), luteinizing hormone (LH) and thyroid stimulating hormone (TSH). All of these hormones are released from the brain and are necessary for ovulation, sex hormone production, energy levels, metabolism, gut function—the list goes on.

Fiber

Fiber is the "meaty" part of fruits and vegetables. It provides food for our microbiome, the good bacteria in the gut. These bacteria help with various functions of the body, including the production of neurotransmitters as well as some vitamins, like vitamin B12. When fruits and vegetables are consumed in their whole forms, which includes the fiber, it helps to minimize blood sugar spikes (one of the other Female Fundamentals).

It's not just about calories though…

Micronutrients

The vitamins and minerals in our foods allow our cells to communicate with each other. For the best results, we should mix up the typical vegetables and fruits we eat and include a healthy mix of nuts and seeds. These foods are highly nutrient-dense. Variety is the key.

In the last chapter, we spoke about how common things like dandruff, stretch marks, and cracks on our tongues can indicate particular nutrient deficiencies. Having a nutrient deficiency isn't as simple as consuming more of the nutrient. Sometimes it occurs because our bodies can't absorb the nutrients, or we have a nutrient imbalance. I often see this in women who experience persistent iron deficiency, even after supplementation or infusion. Oftentimes, as mentioned, the answer lies in them not being able to absorb the nutrients, or having an imbalance in other nutrients like copper, vitamin A, zinc, and manganese, which affects the way they utilize iron.

~

The balance of certain nutrients has been found to contribute to common "diseases" and dysfunctions:

- Low sodium to potassium ratio combined with a high copper to zinc ratio can contribute to dyslexia.[29]
- High calcium to potassium ratio can indicate an underfunctioning thyroid (even if your bloods are "normal"). This can contribute to feelings of bloating, fatigue, dry skin, brain fog, and IBS.
- Low sodium to potassium ratio can also contribute to phobias, panic attacks, indecision, and withdrawal.
- Low calcium to magnesium ratio can contribute to trouble falling asleep, anxiety, and IBS. Calcium has a sedative and calming effect on the nervous system and helps smooth muscle contractility. Not having enough can produce the opposite effect.
- High zinc to copper ratio can contribute to an increased risk of high cholesterol, particularly if consuming too much vitamin C.
- High copper indicates poor liver detoxification and can contribute to higher estrogen levels, PMS, and even those white spots on your fingernails.

If you've been labeled with a diagnosis, or always thought of yourself as an anxious person, or thought that IBS ran in your family, consider that what you're experiencing are messages from your body asking you to help it rebalance.

My favorite way to assess nutrients (and the other three Fundamentals) is through a hair tissue mineral analysis (HTMA) created by Dr. David L. Watts. You'll find more resources about this in the "Resources" section of this book or on our website, www.femalefundamentals.com.au.

How Do You Know You Have a Micronutrient Issue?

Often, you may experience beige flags like stretch marks, dry hair, white spots on your fingernails, chicken skin arms, skin tags, dry cracked mouth, ulcers, or other more significant symptoms, but your blood and medical tests say you're fine.

Things people classically say or experience when consumption is an issue

- "I've tried every diet under the sun."
- "I'm a fussy eater."
- Current or past history of eating disorders.
- Lack variety in their diets. They're "meal prep the same meals each week" type of people.
- Exclude whole food groups.
- "I've been on the same food plan from my gym shred for the past six months."

If you're concerned about what you're putting in or on your body, the general rule is: the closer to nature, the better. Also, when you connect to your body, you'll find that the foods you're craving are often high in the nutrients your body needs.

Always come back to your body, listen to what it's telling you. This doesn't mean, "My body is telling me it's craving a whole block of chocolate and a wheel of cheese." Your body will often give you subtle hints... *Mmmhh, I would really love a margarita right now*. It typically doesn't say, *Mmmmmh, yes, you should have that seventh margarita right now*. At that stage, it's probably talking to you in Spanish. "No más, por favor."

What Should We Avoid?
- Anything that causes inflammation
- Environmental toxins (plastics, home renovations, heavy metals, sprays, fragrances, pesticides)
- Processed foods
- Foods with excipients (common names are soy lecithin, stearic acids, sucrose, sorbitol)
- Alcohol, illicit and medicinal drugs
- Mold
- Cosmetics (fake tans, injectables)
- Big swings in blood sugars

ARE YOU ABSORBING AND UTILIZING YOUR NUTRIENTS?

We can be filling up our bodies with the best of the best nutrients but can sometimes have trouble absorbing them.

You could be like one of my patients, Kate, who suffered with IBS, hyperthyroidism, and inflammation in her body that left her feeling puffy all over. She went through a radical change with her food, cutting out anything ultra-processed and focusing on organic meats and a variety of vegetables and fruits, with healthy fats and carbs included. She also removed toxins in her environment and cosmetics.

Following the changes, she noticed that her puffiness decreased substantially, and her body composition did too. However, she still had issues with her thyroid. Her antibodies were still high, even though she had removed all sources of environmental inflammation. What was missing?

Kate is a chronic people pleaser. She often struggles to make a decision because she's thinking of the 50 other different points of view, constantly living from other people's perspectives and trying to keep everyone else happy. When she does make a decision for herself, she has to quash the guilt she feels because of her perceptions of others' thoughts. People-pleasing tendencies are associated with a fawn response. This isn't a bad response; it served Kate well in the past, training her body to reinforce this behavior because it kept her safe. Only now, the pattern had become so ingrained in her daily life that she was losing sight of herself. When this happens, a couple of things occur in the body.

~~~

The chronic fawn response (red light) triggers the body's metabolism to slow down, decreasing our ability to combat inflammation.

Our stomach acid production decreases so we can't break down foods like we once did, which adds to incoming inflammation. This is what I call the clusterfuck of increased inflammation and a decreased ability to combat the inflammation.

A quick note on inflammation. Inflammation isn't bad. It's part of the process of healing. You can think of it like a light dimmer, instead of a light switch. It's not that it's on or off; it's that we can adapt and have the perfect ambiance of light for our bodies by changing the dimmer and balancing the inflammation coming in with inflammation reduction.

The immune system, like the mind, can sometimes get confused between ourselves and others. Trying to live from the perspective of 50 other people's perceptions is a very confusing and stressful place to live mentally, but it also causes the immune system to become confused between our tissues and other tissues. So, we start to hyper react to our environments, including toxins and foods as well as our own body tissues. In Kate's case, her body started to attack her own thyroid gland because it got confused between self and other.

So, what did she need to work on? Repatterning her people-pleasing tendencies and understanding how to find safety in green lights most of the time.

Things people classically say when absorption is an issue

- "I just react to everything."
- "I get reflux all the time."
- "I'm constantly bloated."

- "I have chronic deficiencies" (for example, iron).
- "I've had a parasite."

Signs of an absorption issue

- Feel tired after eating
- Always hungry
- Bowel urgency
- Bloating
- Painful joints or fogginess in the brain after eating
- Recent history of gastrointestinal infection
- Cracked lips, tongue, or nails

Things that block or affect absorption

- **Halogens**. Fluoride and chlorine are the most common and have been shown to inhibit our thyroid hormones.
- **Hormone-mimicking chemicals**. Fake tans, injectable tans, inhaled tans, and vaping (don't get me started on vaping!) all expose us to substances that mimic our own hormones, making it difficult for our bodies to find balance.
- **Heavy metals**. Heavy metals often antagonize nutrients. Lead is known to block calcium, and mercury to compete with iron, zinc, selenium, and sulfur.
- **Oral contraceptives**. Because we consume them orally, oral contraceptives can affect the gut's ability to absorb nutrients by affecting mucus within the gut. As a result, absorbing nutrients, such as B vitamins, magnesium, zinc,

and CoQ10, becomes more difficult.[30] Our guts weren't designed to interact with hormones in this way.

Are There Such Things as Good or Bad Foods?

Have you ever known someone to react to pretty much anything? They could eat a $120 organic rib eye steak and still get IBS. Surely, a food that humans have been eating for generations couldn't be causing the body to react like this... When we experience reactions to foods that are "good," or have been known as food to humans for many generations, it often comes down to two possibilities. Has the manufacturing process altered the food so our bodies can't recognize it like it once did? Or... are our digestive systems having trouble digesting it?

Different parts of the digestive system are designed to digest different components of food. For instance, our mouths secrete saliva, which houses an enzyme called amylase that helps to break down simple carbohydrates. Our chewing also helps to break down the structure of our food and prime our guts for what's about to be sent down farther.

Our stomachs have stomach acid and enzymes that help to digest proteins. The upper part of the small intestine houses the junction where bile meets pancreatic enzymes, which help to digest fats, and more complex carbohydrates are digested farther down the small intestine. If our bodies are struggling to produce acids, enzymes, or bile in these areas, the food can pass along in a partially undigested form. This can create reactions in different parts of the gut because they're not used to "seeing" that type of food, which explains why sometimes you can eat a food and not react, and other times you eat the same food have a reaction. Or why you're bloating or having reactions to multiple whole foods.

Sometimes it's the food pretending to be something it's not and catfishing you. Sometimes it's your body trying to tell you something.

~~~

When intermittent fasting first came into vogue (do people still say vogue?), I was eager to try it. I did time-restricted eating, having an eating window between 12 p.m. and 8 p.m., with a 16-hour window of no food. This was designed to reduce inflammation, reduce hunger hormones, and boost overall health.

After doing it for around four weeks, my skin was breaking out; I was agitated, and I had gained weight. What I didn't take into consideration was my Female Fundamentals. I wasn't eating enough protein in my eating window; my stress levels were high due to work demands at the time, and I wasn't getting enough variety in my nutrients. In this instance, the fasting was "too much" stress on my body. I didn't have the right balance of internal resources to meet the demand I was putting on it, so my body started to tell me through my skin, moods, and weight that it wasn't happy.

Always use your body as the guide, even when society is telling you something different.

What About Supplements?

What I've seen from my patients is that those who rely solely on supplements as the "magic fix" notice their symptoms return when they cease using them—and for good reason. They're still trying to achieve balance with their Female Fundamentals, but they're not quite there yet. The people who have the best results are those who make changes to integrate the 4 Female Fundamentals into their lives while on the supplements. The Female Fundamentals are the cake; the supplements are the cherries on top.

When we have a chronic imbalance in our nutrients, we often feel crap. Trying to make changes to your lifestyle when you feel like your body is running on empty is extremely hard, no matter how much willpower you have. However, when your body is supported with the specific supplements it needs, it's like your car (from the earlier analogy) starts running again. It's difficult to feel like you can get back on track when your car (body) struggles to even start.

The trick is, once your car starts, you need to work to change your lifestyle so you don't continue down the same 4WD track. If you're driving a Ferrari, that lifestyle simply isn't suited to your car.

Can You Excrete Toxins? (Exhaust)

Our bodies detoxify through the gut, liver and gallbladder, urine, sweat, lymphatics, menstrual cycle, breath, skin, and sleep. If you're noticing issues with any of these systems, your body is telling you it needs you to support your detoxification.

When we don't support detoxification, things like heavy metals, excess hormones, environmental hormone mimics, and inflammation can increase in the body. Like a car, we need the exhaust to excrete our bodies' by-products.

How do you know if you have an excretion issue?

Several symptoms can indicate an issue with excretion:

- Acne
- Cellulite
- Bloating
- Constipation (not going at least once a day)
- Fluid retention
- Aching joints
- Immobility throughout the day
- Glands always seem "to be up"
- Poor sleep
- Chronic adenoid, sinus, or tonsillitis inflammation
- Loss of menstrual cycle (premenopause)

How can you support excretion?

Firstly, identify the source of toxins to stop exposure. Common forms of exposure I've seen in patients include sleeping next to a partner who is a heavy smoker (this has been shown to affect egg quality too[31]), soil and air pollution, amalgam fillings, heavy metals in water supply (look for discoloration around your taps, or have you water checked if you're concerned), crop sprays, cosmetics, and work environments (welding, plumbing, farming, and so on). If you want to know for sure what your levels are, a HTMA test can be a great place to start.

The second step is to increase your nutrition and hydration. The better your nutrition, the better nutrients will bind and excrete toxins.

Thirdly, ensure your elimination pathways are open. Pooping once a day, massaging your lymph nodes, dry brushing, regular menstrual cycles, having great sleep, and moving your body for at least 30 minutes a day is helpful for almost everyone.

How Can You Measure Your Nutrients?

The thing we always have to remember with nutrients is that the body is one smart cookie. Just like the mum I mentioned earlier with the toddler snacks, our bodies like to store and have nutrients on hand, just in case of emergency.

What this looks like is the main nutrients our cells use to help our bodies function are either in circulation (snacks given to the toddler now) or stored in body tissues, like our bones and organs (snacks in the handbag, just in case).

Largely, when we check our nutrient levels on blood tests, we're checking what's in our serum, meaning, how many snacks does our toddler have? The number of snacks the toddler has depends on how the mum is deciding to divvy up her resources.

To check reserve levels in the tissues, a HTMA can be used. This helps us understand what snacks mum has in reserve and the overall function of her thinking. (Is it dinner time in an hour? Have they had enough protein for the day? Shit, we've had the same meal for the last three nights in a row… Have the kids been at the beach all day running around? They probably need some extra snacks before dinner). Our bodies are also asking questions. (Are we sick? Have we had enough sleep? Is our relationship falling to shambles? Are we running a marathon? Is it hot outside?).

Mums, like our bodies, are super smart. They're always considering how much they have in reserve and how much they should give now. It's probably why my mum still asks if anyone is hungry and always has the fridge and cupboard stocked with food, even though my siblings and I are all old enough to get food ourselves. Who doesn't love a stocked fridge though?

So, when a blood test is abnormal, it means the kids either have too many snacks or not enough. The body, aka Mum, isn't realizing that the reserves of snacks are low and it doesn't have enough money (intake) to buy more. If the levels are high, Mum might be a little sleep-deprived and forget that she's already given you your third snack and it's not even lunchtime yet. Either way, there's something wrong with Mum (the body's ability to balance).

This is why it's important to look not just at medical testing for nutrients but also functional testing.

～

Remember Maeve from Chapter 2? At age 21, she was told she'd be on thyroid medication her whole life, based on what her blood tests told us. After looking at her functional health, we found on her HTMA that her arsenic levels were high; she was also low in the nutrients her body needed to respond to her thyroid hormone. After three months of using the 4 Female Fundamentals to guide her lifestyle and replacing specific nutrients, her thyroid function improved, and her blood test returned to normal, without needing to go on thyroid medication.

How Can You Support Your Nutrients?

As a starting point, supporting the other three Female Fundamentals is always going to support your nutrients. If you've identified that you need primary support for your nutrients, you can try the following steps.

Remove exposure to negative nutrients

Alcohol, vaping, drug use, sources of hormone mimickers, fragrances, emulsifiers (commonly substances like soy lecithin).

Add exposure to positive nutrients

Variety is key here—a balance of protein, fat, and carbs as well as fruit, vegetables, nuts, and seeds.

Improve absorption

Supporting your nervous system will greatly support gut function and absorption. Chew your food and if you're prone to bloating in the mornings, boost bitter foods and supplement with digestive enzymes if you wish.

Improve excretion

Prioritize sleep, massage your lymph nodes, boost pooping to at least once per day, breathe, get enough good nutrients in, hydrate, boost sulfur-rich foods like seafood, beans, nuts, and seeds for liver function.

Nutrients and Emotions

The raw materials of our bodies largely impact our moods. We know that when we're hungry and have low blood sugar, we can feel agitated, and when we eat, the agitation goes away. Alcoholics know this too. When they consume alcohol, it helps to sedate and numb their minds. Even if you're not an alcoholic but enjoy the occasional glass, you know it's going to affect your mood. We can alter our moods and emotions by changing our body chemistry.

If you experience more consistent emotional patterns, like phobias, anxiety, depression, repression, and panic attacks, they're often not in your head or a default pattern but, again, a reflection of your internal mineral state and external environment. Often, for example, low calcium is linked to increased states of anxiety, and high calcium is linked to depression. This is because of the sedative nature of the mineral. Imbalances of sodium and potassium can impact comprehension and mental clarity. Just as we can change our moods through the impact of food or alcohol on our nutrients, our moods can be altered because of our baseline internal nutrients.

Your moods are not in your head. They're in your body.

Calories in, Calories out

The reason why your diet is no longer working and you're gaining weight isn't because you need to reduce your calories even more.

It's because you need to support your body. Think about it really simply. If you previously did one thing and it gave you a certain output, and you did the same thing, but it gave you a different output, is it the thing that you haven't changed (the calories) or could something else have changed?

It's not the calories that have changed; it's that your body has.

It's like putting 100 g of pasta into a boiling pot of water versus putting 100 g of pasta in the cupboard. Same input, different output. Your body is either the pot of boiling water or the cupboard. What makes you a pot of boiling water or the cupboard are your Female Fundamentals.

Looking for the Best Diet? You're not Alone

A common question I get asked is, "What's the best diet?" The short answer: a diet, much like a diagnosis, just makes it easier for us to explain to others what type of food we can and cannot eat.

Your body doesn't care what you call it; it just cares if you can give it what it needs. Your food should aim to provide the building blocks your body needs to function, balance blood sugars, and limit inflammation. In order to do this, some general guidelines apply:

Variety

Variety in our macro and micronutrients helps provide the building blocks of essential functions in our bodies. If you're limiting variety, you're likely limiting your ability to function.

Blood sugars

Having a balance of proteins, fats, and carbohydrates helps achieve stable blood sugars. You'll see specific tips in the blood sugar section of this chapter.

Eat food that is food

The more processed it is, the more likely it is to create inflammation in your body. Aim to reduce packages and plastics.

~

It seems like every 2–3 years, there's a new diet or eating regiment that promises to be the magic cure we've been looking for. Typically, however, a good diet comes down to the level of inflammation it's going to cause, whether our blood sugars remain relatively balanced, we receive a wide variety of nutrients, as well as a low toxic load on the body (if your liver and lymphatics will be able to process it).

Here are a few examples:

Fasting—Helps with inflammation and blood sugar regulation.

Keto—Helps with inflammation and blood sugars.

Carnivore—Limits possibility of inflammatory foods and assists with blood sugar regulation.

Vegan—Possibly helps with inflammation but depends on the type of vegan and the foods that enter the body.

Ultimately, we can achieve balanced blood sugars, low inflammation, and variety in our nutrients by caring for all four of our Female Fundamentals. A diet can be a helpful tool, but it's not the diet—it's what the diet is aiming to achieve—that makes the impact.

Quiz on Nutrients

If you want to find out what nutrients need support, take the free Female Fundamentals quiz on our website: www.femalefundamentals.com.au/resources.

BLOOD SUGARS

The two modes of your Hybrid car. Which fuel mode are you using?

Blood sugars are part of our energy regulation, which has two modes, much like a hybrid car. We have the sugar in our blood, the fuel that's easily activated and used in the bloodstream, and the stored fuel in the battery, in the form of fat in our liver, muscles, and adipose tissue. We can use the fuel coming in, which in this case is blood sugars. Or we can use our stored fuel (battery charge), which in the case of our bodies is ketones. This is what we use when we're in a fasted state.

When we have fuel coming in consistently, our bodies get used to using our fuel. When we have an excess amount of fuel, our blood sugars can rise too high. Remember, our bodies are all about balance. When this happens, the body does this tricky thing where it pulls some of those blood sugars into the muscles and liver to be stored. Once they start to fill up, we then hide any excess sugar that's in the blood in our fat cells. When this happens over and over, it causes our fat cells to swell, get larger; hence, our body fat increases.

Whether or not our bodies are using the fuel from our fuel lines (blood sugars) or the fuel from our stored battery (fat) is dependent on the presence of insulin.

What Causes Insulin to be Released?

Think of your blood sugars like turning your garden hose on and filling up a bucket with sugary water. This bucket needs to always have just the right amount of water in it, and the role of your insulin is to make sure the water level is just right. If it's not, the sugary water goes everywhere, which is bad for your body, triggering widespread inflammation, damage to nerves, heart, kidneys, eyes, and nervous system, hormone imbalance, increased anxiety, immune system weakening, damage to our cells, and, in severe cases, diabetic coma. Thankfully, your body has some tricks up its sleeve to balance these levels and keep the sugary water from rising too high and overflowing or going too low.

When the sugary water is trickling into the bucket, it's easy for insulin to come along with a sponge and mop it up. The first sponges that fill up are the liver and muscles, which is why high blood sugars contribute to fatty liver disease. When we have more muscle mass, we have a bigger sponge for insulin to store glucose. When the liver and muscle sponges fill up, our fat cell sponge starts to fill up and get bigger and bigger and bigger. The more water it needs to mop up, the bigger the sponge gets.

The key to regulating our blood sugars is to give our bodies a break by turning off the tap of sugary water. When this happens, our bodies, like a hybrid car, switch from using fuel in the fuel lines to the stored battery fuel because the bucket isn't threatening to overflow. Instead, the levels are dropping too low. To keep a healthy level of sugary water, the liver and muscle sponges need to squeeze some of their juice into the bucket. As the bucket continues to empty throughout the day, our liver and muscle cells run out of stored fuel so our bodies begin to wring out our fat sponges.

If, at any stage, the sugary water tap turns back on—by consuming carbohydrates, sugary drinks, and, to a lesser degree, proteins—the sponges stop wringing and begin soaking up the water again.

If we eat high-carbohydrate foods, the tap is turned on at high pressure. If the tap is left on at this rate, over time, the sponges reach their limit, and the sugary water leaks out into the rest of the body, causing widespread inflammation and cell damage. Is it any wonder we get skin breakouts, crappy sleep, and moodiness when we've eaten like a kid at a birthday party?

The key to supporting this system is eating food that has a good balance of carbohydrates, fats, and proteins so the water pressure is just right and not bombarding your sponges. We can also support our blood sugar balance by turning off the tap occasionally. Turning off the tap means having a rest period from food intake for at least 12–14 hours. For people who have sponges that are full, with sugary water leaking everywhere, having longer periods of time without the tap on may be beneficial.

~

When we become insulin resistant, it means our liver, muscle, and fat cells have been bombarded by the sugary water for so long that they don't want to soak up anymore, even though our bodies are still trying to tell them to do so. In this case, we see both high blood sugar and high insulin levels.

In the case of diabetics who can't produce insulin (the hormone that tells our sponges to soak up the water), their bodies effectively don't know how to get the water into the sponges, so they need medication to help them know when to mop it up.

The sponges can become resistant to the messages from the body telling them to soak up the sugary water for a number of reasons:

- **Overload**. Sponges are already full due to chronic overeating or exposure to repetitive blood sugar spikes.
- **Poor sleep.** Upsetting the circadian rhythm confuses the body, and sponges don't know if they should be soaking up or wringing out.
- **Environmental toxins.** These can damage the cells of the pancreas that produce insulin.
- **Nutrient deficiency.** Chromium, manganese, calcium, and magnesium are important in insulin regulation.
- **Nutrient excess.** Excess iron as well as cobalt have been found to damage the cells of the pancreas that produce insulin.

- **Brain hormone signals.** High levels of stress-released cortisol trigger more sugary water pressure and decrease the sponge's ability to absorb it.
- **Inflammation.** Inflammation increases insulin levels, and high insulin levels trigger inflammation. This often causes a vicious loop that makes it difficult to lose weight.

Blood Sugars, Fat, and Weight Loss Loop

When our blood sugars rise, so does inflammation. High blood sugar means insulin is released to bring it down. The blood sugar levels decrease because insulin has hidden the sugar in our fatty tissue. Our fatty tissue also raises inflammation. When inflammation rises, so do our blood sugars. This can make it difficult to lose weight when we're inflamed and insulin-resistant.

Signs of insulin resistance

You can have insulin resistance without having the physical signs, but you may have:

- Weight gain around the upper body and around the middle
- Skin tags
- Fatty liver
- Acanthosis nigricans (skin discoloration in the creases of your body)
- Hangry episodes
- Mood swings
- Dizziness without food

- Sweet-smelling breath
- Unquenchable thirst
- Sleep apnea

Blood tests to detect insulin resistance

- High triglycerides
- High cholesterol
- Elevated ALT
- Elevated CRP
- HbA1c—how much water has leaked over the pavement and into the rest of the body over the last three months
- Fasting insulin
- Glucose tolerance test with insulin

How Do Blood Sugars Link to the Other Fundamentals?

Nervous system

We know that when the nervous system is in an orange light, it needs more sugar in the blood to have access to quick energy, which causes our insulin levels to go down. We also know that when we give a perfectly calm child sugar, they can become a lot less calm. We've moved them from a green light to an orange light, purely through the blood sugar spike we've given them. It's also why when you start your morning with a bowl of sugary cereal and a coffee, you drive to work feeling anxious, compared to when you start it with a couple of eggs and avocado.

Metabolism

Diabetics will know that they need to pay attention to their blood sugars more when they come down with a cold or infection. We know that illness, whether chronic or acute, alters our metabolism. An increased metabolism requires higher blood sugars, and a slowed metabolism often results in an increase in sugar storage in the liver and adipose tissue. Metabolic flexibility is our ability to switch between burning glucose and burning fat, the two modes of the hybrid car, and that is the ideal.

Nutrients

Macronutrients like carbohydrates boost blood sugars quickly. However, protein doesn't boost them to the same degree, and fats don't trigger a spike in blood sugars at all, although they can affect blood sugars by making it more difficult for your body to reduce them. Micronutrients like calcium, magnesium, chromium, and manganese aid in the release of insulin and your body's sensitivity to it.

They all trigger and support each other.

Stress and Poor Sleep

A patient who is in her early 30s, super fit, and a gym owner competes in national level fitness competitions. She eats a clean diet, with a great balance of macros and creates a calorie deficit when wanting to lose weight. Except she finds it difficult to lose weight and if she does lose any, it always comes back on.

Her blood tests signify that her fasting glucose is on the brink at 5.4 mmol/L (top of the range is 5.5 mmol/L). In her case, she's seemingly controlling the pressure of the water coming into the bucket, but the level is getting into more dangerous territory.

So, what's happening with her?

It seems like her stress levels, poor sleep, and lack of sunlight in the morning are contributing to her increased water pressure (blood glucose), as well as her body not being as sensitive to soaking up the sugary water with her sponges.

She also eats late at night, so her sponges don't have much time to wring out into the bucket.

How did we help her?

- Supported her nervous system and nutrients by supporting her adrenal glands with herbs and minerals that replenished them. Also prioritized rest and connection with friends.
- Supported her metabolism by creating an eating window of 8–10 hours—to give her body time to wring out the sponges overnight—and also limited blue light and boosted sunlight.

Since making the changes, she has noticed slow and progressive weight loss, along with boosted energy levels, restful sleep, and decreased inflammation.

How to Support Your Blood Sugars

You'll see that your other Female Fundamentals are infused in the tips below.

Control the tap pressure of the sugary water

- Eat around 1.5–2 g of protein per kg of body weight or up to 150 g (or 5.3 oz) of protein per day. At the very least, ensure that you have protein as a component of each meal.
- Avoid ultra-processed foods.
- Avoid high-dose fructose (soft drinks, desserts, fruit juices).
- Boost oxytocin through pleasure and play, and reduce stress.
- As Jessie Inchauspé, the "Glucose Goddess," has found, having vinegar before your meals, as well as consuming your food in order (salad and non-starchy veggies, proteins and fats, then starches like pasta and rice), can significantly reduce the glucose spike—that is, sugary water pressure.[32]

Help your sponges wring

- **Build muscle.** This boosts insulin sensitivity and creates a bigger sponge for the sugary water to "hide" in.
- **Move your body after eating.**
- **Time-restricted eating.** Enables the sugary water to stop and the sponges to wring water back into the bucket to restore balance.

Help your body know whether to wring or soak (insulin sensitivity)

- Reduce inflammation by minimizing inflammatory foods and supporting the nervous system.
- Support healthy circadian rhythm with morning light and eating at similar times every day.

- Get enough sleep.
- Assess which micronutrients your body may need (best way is through a functional HTMA test).
- Switching to a temporary low-carb or keto diet can be good for severe insulin resistance.
- Maintain a healthy menstrual cycle (by supporting your Female Fundamentals).
- Women may want to minimize testosterone-based contraceptives because too much testosterone can reduce insulin sensitivity.

The fine balance of sugary water in the bucket (blood sugars) is maintained by balancing these three main factors.

Quiz on Blood Sugars

If you want to find out if your blood sugars need support, take the free Female Fundamentals quiz on our website: www.femalefundamentals.com.au/resources.

HOW DO THE FUNDAMENTALS RELATE TO EACH OTHER? IS ONE MORE IMPORTANT THAN THE OTHER?

My grandma was the type of person who was ahead of her time. She made her own kombucha before anyone had ever heard about it. She had her own colloidal silver machine and even though she left school when she was 14, she became a naturopath when she was in her early 50s. She was always mixing up different potions for us when we got sick. She taught me many amazing things, least of which was that the body is always giving us the clues we need to know how to help it. The other was that no matter how well you looked after your body, if stress was involved, it would trump everything.

My grandma died from congestive heart failure when she was 76. Even though she took great care of the nutrients she put in and on her body (she was known for using her own urine for skincare), had amazing friends and family connections, enjoyed painting as well as exercising and being out in nature, her body fell apart.

In the small town I grew up in, everyone knew my grandma. When patients found out she was my grandma, they often offered the same remark: "Oh, Carol, she was a saint. She was so lovely, and a bit cheeky too!"

She *was* a saint; she cared for everyone around her so deeply and would often say to my mum, "Be like a duck. Calm on the surface and paddling like crazy below." I think about this often and wonder whether that was her undoing. Doing for others and caring for others more than she cared for herself. Maybe she needed a little less saint and a little more cheekiness. Maybe we all do.

We Need to Stop Thinking of Our Bodies in Silos

You might think that you don't think of your body in a silo. You know that everything is connected. You know the importance of things like fasting and breathwork, and you practically have a PhD in health podcasts and books (including this one). Understanding that everything is connected is one thing; actually connecting to your body is another.

When we're in connection with our bodies, we can use them as our guides to know what to do for them, instead of adhering to the latest trends or the demands of our lives. Just because you booked in that early morning spin class, it doesn't mean you're flaky, a terrible friend, or a fat lazy b*tch if you decide not to go. It's not just about will power. Did you change your mind? Or were you just listening to your body?

A simple thing you can do is, when you wake up in the morning, get in the practice of connecting with your body. Once you've connected to it, ask it, *What do you need right now?*

It might say, *I need you to get up and go to that spin class, we need to move.* Or it might say, *We need another hour's rest.* Or it might say, *You need to go for a walk in the sunshine, or do some yoga, give yourself a hug, get up and dance naked, or sit and read with a cup of tea.*

Our bodies tell us what we need, but we often override them with feelings of guilt for not following through on what we previously said we would do, the perceived demands of our lives. Or we feel shame—because what would people think? What kind of person would you be if you changed your mind?

You always have permission to change your mind, especially when your body is telling you to do so.

When we focus on the next health trend being our savior, it reinforces the pattern of treating our bodies in silos and out of context.

Breathwork isn't for everyone and not for everyone all of the time. Same with ice baths and the keto diet and fasting and veganism.

Basically, I don't care how you achieve the 4 Female Fundamentals. It could be momentarily through one of these trends—they're helpful for a reason—but when we become too attached to a particular trend, we can start to use it to make decisions for us, and we can become deaf to our bodies.

Chronic disease happens when we choose our minds over our bodies over and over again.

~~~

Let's meet one of my patients, Mary, who, at the bottom of her first history form, wrote, *Help me please!*

She's a 48-year-old who has been experiencing a plethora of symptoms her whole life. Ranging from persistent fatigue, weight gain (even though she had been exercising and limiting her calories), a history of cysts on her ovaries, endometriosis, and she would describe herself as a people pleaser. Even after seeing multiple doctors, specialists, and alternative practitioners, no one was able to find anything on her tests, so she was told there was nothing wrong with her. This, understandably, left her feeling deflated and hopeless. She'd tried everything she knew, and now she was asking for help and wasn't able to find it. She was making all the shifts, minimizing her calories, upping her strength and fat burning training, but still nothing was shifting.

When we dug a little deeper, she also reported experiencing brain fog, memory issues, fatigue, dry skin, depression, insomnia, headaches, and anxiety. At first, she didn't think to mention these because she'd been experiencing them for such a long time, consistently being told there was nothing wrong on her blood tests. So, she considered her symptoms "normal." It was time to change that.

We implemented all 4 Female Fundamentals into her life, because they all impact each other. Let's see if you can spot them…

We increased protein throughout her day, swapping her breakfast for one with more protein and fat. We also brought in a 30-minute walk every day and swapped her weight training to four times a week in the afternoons, which removed the stress of getting up in a rush to lift weights, helping her be in green lights in the mornings and minimizing blood sugar spikes. Instead, she switched to drinking a cup of tea, listening to music in the morning sun (extra tick for the sun), and strengthening the connection between her and her body (you'll learn more about this in the next chapter). We also incorporated specific supplementation to bring balance to her mineral profile, helping to boost her adrenal, thyroid, and metabolic function.

I saw her for our three-month checkup, and she looked like a completely different person. She was quite literally glowing. I jokingly asked her if she was pregnant—she wasn't. Her smile was brighter, and I could sense, even through the screen, that she had more energy and vibrance. Her face even looked less puffy.

However, she wasn't over the moon like I thought she would be. She said, "I'm feeling so much better, I can think clearly, I have energy, my sex life is back, and I've lost 3 kilos ... But what I'm worried about is that this is just a fluke and I'll go back to how I *really* am."

This broke my heart. What Mary didn't realize was that this was her ... *really*. This was how her body was built to work. We had finally given it what it needed so she started feeling different. Just as her body felt different when she wasn't giving it what it needed. It was never her body. She was never broken. Her body was giving her the answers all along.

When we have the mindset and understanding that our body knows what to do, all we have to do is give it what it needs and then move the fuck out of the way.

~~~

You might be experiencing something similar to Mary, or a mixture of your own symptoms. Running around trying to fix the headaches and then the hormone imbalance and PMS and the IBS and the chronic weakened immune system... It can be confusing as fuck to be a woman, with people from every direction telling you something different. All we want is to understand what our bodies need, give it to them, feel amazing, and be able to live our lives the way we want to.

> **One of the ways people might get sick and unhappy is by continually following through on things that are out of alignment with their bodies.**

We're constantly looking outside of ourselves for the miracle fix when, really, our bodies are the miracle—we just need to get out of the way.

Putting Them All Together

People often ask me, "Which Fundamental is the most important?" The short answer is: all of them are equally important.

The long answer, however…

Our bodies are mirrors. They reflect back to us how we're maintaining balance between our inner and outer world. We do this through all four of our Female Fundamentals.

I'll give you an example. When you're stressed, what food choices do you make?

When you're calm, what food choices do you make? How do you respond to someone cutting you off in traffic if you haven't had sleep or you're hungry? What about if you've had an amazing sleep and you're full?

The actions we take are based on the balance of all four of our Female Fundamentals. All of them are important in the system.

**What all of the health fads, biohacks,
and tips for improving your health have in
common are—the 4 Female Fundamentals.**

Remember, it's not about the fasting, the breathwork, the sleep, the carnivore, keto, or raw juice. Forget about the magical fix. Remember your body. Your body doesn't care about marketing, about what's hot right now. It cares about having what it fundamentally needs.

You'll find simple breakdowns of the "hottest new health trends" and how they stack up to the Female Fundamentals on our online platforms—link in the resource section of the book.

4 Female Fundamentals and Your Hormones

A common question I get asked is, "What about my hormones? Are they balanced or not?" Often, they've looked up all the signs of estrogen dominance or high testosterone and have concluded that's what they have, but it's not always that simple.

Our hormones are a constant moving target, as is everything in the body. They adapt depending on what signals our bodies are receiving. When we're told we have a hormone imbalance, like estrogen dominance or high cortisol, it's important to understand why it's happening. Knowing what's going on isn't enough; we need to dig deeper and understand why our bodies are adapting in that way. By now you know, when I'm talking about why, I'm talking about the Female Fundamentals.

"I get serious fluctuations in my symptoms when my hormones change."

Imagine these fluctuations across the month like the ocean. There are always going to be waves that come and go and tides that rise and fall. This is natural; it's healthy; it's necessary to create our hormones. After a while, we learn to surf these waves.

What happens to the waves if one day the seabed floor shifts from an earthquake? No longer are they the waves we learned to surf; they're tsunamis that can leave us feeling like we're drowning. We experience debilitating hot flashes, insomnia, rage, intense food cravings, fatigue, brain fog, pain, headaches, weight gain, immune challenges, anxiety, and gut changes. The seabed floor is your Female Fundamentals. When we ground in the Fundamentals of the body, the seabed is stable; it's strong; it doesn't shake, even though the tides are always changing.

It's normal to feel more exhilarated at some points in your cycle, like when you catch a wave of progesterone and estrogen around ovulation, and it's normal to feel a lull between sets when your hormone levels have dropped and your bleed arrives. But if you feel like you're drowning, it's likely that the Fundamentals have become shaky, causing the waves to become more difficult to surf. Think about your hormones like the rest of your body, as a mirror of the 4 Fundamentals.

Most oral contraceptives work by turning the waves into a lake, removing the ebbs and flows of natural hormone production. When the contraceptives are stopped, the waves return. How you feel when you stop oral contraceptives depends on the size of the waves—your 4 Female Fundamentals, your seabed floor.

Women's hormones also change across their lifespans. This is like learning to surf a new beach. We experience a new beach around the "great magnifiers" of puberty, pregnancy, postpartum, and perimenopause. If you're struggling with symptoms around these stages, you need to tweak how you're looking after your Female Fundamentals. This is why some women breeze through puberty, pregnancy, postpartum, and perimenopause, and others don't. Contrary to what we've been conditioned to think, it's not because some women are unlucky or broken, or that it's out of her control. It has to do with their Fundamentals.

The main thing to remember—ride the waves. If you feel like you're holding on for dear life, those waves have turned into tsunamis, and you need to focus on your Fundamentals. Like when one month you're an absolute mess when your period arrives, and the next you're not too bad. One month your Fundamentals were balanced, and you could surf the wave when it came, and the other month you were out of your depth.

CAN MEN USE THE 4 FEMALE FUNDAMENTALS?

Since implementing this framework with female patients, I often get the question, "Can this also help my brother, partner, dad, husband, friend?" The short answer is *yes*. This framework is applicable to men, and I've had many men have success with it. "Male Mundamentals" just doesn't quite have the same ring to it.

TOP 10 FOR YOUR FEMALE FUNDAMENTALS

#1. Start your day getting into the green traffic light

Notice how you feel when you wake up. Are you already in a rush? Do you feel tired and drowsy? Get into the green light by connecting to a sense of calm, pleasure, play, curiosity—whatever that means for you. I personally love to put on some music for whichever emotion I want to feel and move my body in that way. Typically, it's dancing naked in my room.

#2. Connect to your body like it's your number one job

When we connect to our bodies, we make decisions that are in alignment with what our body needs. It also makes connecting with others easier.

#3. Breathe

Just as our breath changes when we're stressed, we can change our breath to alter how the nervous system feels.

#4. Light

Expose yourself to sunlight within the first and last couple hours of the day. This supports your metabolism and circadian rhythm. Rhythm is what aids in the overall balance of our bodies.

#5. Magnetism

Put your bare feet on the earth and soak yourself in nature. This helps your body balance your energy levels. Particularly how your mitochondria create energy.

#6. Minimize the crap

Minimize crap food, crap people, crap thoughts. We find this easier when we care for our Fundamentals and our capacity increases.

#7. Balance your blood sugars

When eating, aim for nutrient variety (both macro and micro) and balancing blood sugars—I don't care what "diet" you subscribe to.

#8. Give your body what it needs

Hint—it's hard to know what that is when we haven't done #1 and #2. The more you do this, the stronger the connection and trust you build with yourself. Remembering that what your body needs are your Fundamentals, you can objectively test these via the "test your fundamentals" on our website and find resources to support your Fundamentals here too.

#9. Move your body

This helps remove toxins, balance blood sugars, regulate your nervous system, and support your metabolism.

#10. Check your Fundamentals

When you're considering a change due to a health fad, ask yourself, *How does it stack up with the Fundamentals?* You'll find breakdowns of common health trends and your Fundamentals on our website.

A GUIDE: WHAT THE FEMALE FUNDAMENTALS LOOK LIKE IN ACTION

It's not so much that you need to add more things into your day; it's more about making the things you're already doing Female-Fundamentals-friendly.

Use them as a guide to know what your body needs at any given time.

You're eating breakfast? Make it Female Fundamentals friendly by making it high in proteins and fats.

You're exercising? Make it Female Fundamentals friendly by doing it in a non-stressed state, or moving after food.

You're waking up? Make waking up a green light by giving yourself time to connect to your body.

You're hanging out with friends? Be present and connect to release oxytocin and reduce cortisol.

You're stressed on your way to work? Switch off the podcast and play your favorite song to dance to.

Don't let your mind convince you that better health is going to come from the next magic pill, the next magic diet or the next biohack. Better health comes from listening to what your body needs and giving it the Fundamentals.

To know which of your Female Fundamentals need support, take the free Female Fundamentals quiz and check out our social media and online tools. You'll find links at the back of this book.

So, now that you know that your body talks to you through your symptoms and tells you what it needs to balance your 4 Female Fundamentals, where do you want to go? What do you want?

> ~ *More energy?*
> ~ *To lose weight?*
> ~ *Clear skin?*
> ~ *A healthy relationship to food?*
> ~ *To be pain-free?*
> ~ *Regular periods?*
> ~ *A stronger immune system?*
> ~ *Your libido back?*

We can give our bodies everything they need to function but if we don't pay attention to where we're going, we could be sending them right back down the same bumpy road to get banged up again, and again, and again! You could be driving a Ferrari and sending it down a 4WD track. Pretty soon, that well-functioning car starts to get damaged. Just like it did before you started implementing the changes. This is what happens when you've done everything for your physical body—you're a badass at the Female Fundamentals—but you feel like there's something still holding you back, or you keep repeating old unconscious patterns. This relates to your GPS.

Now that you're an expert on the Female Fundamentals, the final piece of the puzzle is to be conscious about where you want to go…

Chapter 5

ENERGETIC LAYER

~

What we can't see creates what we can see.

STUCK IN PATTERNS

When patients begin medical and functional healing, I often notice two patterns arise that let me know that their energetic health needs some support too. Either they've experienced amazing changes with their health after implementing the Female Fundamentals but feel like they're still band-aiding themselves, or they struggle to notice long-term change because their old patterns have been so heavily ingrained. Sometimes, no matter how much we change, our patterns keep replaying.

This is where the final layer of our health spectrum comes in: our energetics.

I like to think that our energetics are our cars' GPSs. When we can connect to them and follow their guidance, our bodies and our health are in alignment, and we feel alive.

A LITTLE SCIENCE LESSON

Like Wi-Fi, Bluetooth, or music, things that we can't see can impact us greatly. The same is true for our bodies.

The science of the body has largely been focused on evolutionary biology, and only recently has more attention been placed on biophysics. You can think of biology as how the building blocks of our bodies (cells) respond and adapt for our survival, and biophysics as looking at each component of our cells and how they interact with even smaller particles; atoms, neutrons, protons, and electrons. These smaller particles generate a charge, much like the energy that runs your fridge. Everything, from the chair you're sitting on, your body, the air, plants, even your fart, contains energy because it's made up of particles that hold a charge. Whether you know it or not, the vibrational frequency of these particles alters the energy they emit. This frequency then alters what types of tissues it can affect. How does this happen?

What we often don't realize is that there are many energies at play. For instance, we have the energy of visible light from the sun that we can see, and we have UV light, which our eyes cannot register, but it still affects our bodies. We know this because we get sunburned. It's the same reason we can hear certain sounds and others can't. The frequency of the sound is different.

Like sound and UV light, our emotions are also invisible energy that vibrates at different frequencies. We can't see them, but our bodies can feel them.

Signs your energetics may be running unconscious loops

- You notice physical ailments when a significant emotional event happens—for example, your lower back aches when you feel unsupported.
- Every time, at the same time of year, you develop a painful, stiff neck.
- That rash on your body started when you had that huge fight with your partner.
- You're faced with two decisions in life, unsure which way to go, and end up with vertigo (dizziness).
- You're doing something that you know isn't the right thing for you, and you end up with indigestion or heartburn.
- You experience jaw problems when you haven't spoken your truth to someone.
- You unconsciously choose behaviors that are harmful.

My kinesiologist and dear friend once said to me, "When we use our mind to make decisions, we use our body as a resource. When we use our body to make decisions, we use our mind as a resource." What I've found is that the energetic layer of our bodies is linked to our ability to connect to our bodies and use them as our guides. In order to do this, we must be able to connect to and trust our bodies.

CONNECTING TO YOUR BODY (GPS)

So, how do you know when you're using your body or your mind to make a decision?

I had a patient several years ago, let's call her Sandra. She was in her late 40s and was experiencing some persistent lower abdominal pain, which she was worried about. She mentioned it to her husband, who happened to be a healthcare practitioner, as was she. He said, "Oh, don't worry about it, nothing to stress about." She then went and asked her doctor about it, and they said the same thing.

A couple of weeks went by, and she still had this nagging feeling that something wasn't right, so she went to a different doctor in a different town and insisted on getting a scan of her abdomen. What they found was an 8 cm (3 inch) growth that was moments away from turning cancerous.

As mentioned, Sandra is a health practitioner herself—a damn good one at that—and even she had pushback from other practitioners, her partner, and doctors. Had she trusted them more than herself, who knows what would have happened? Did the other doctors and her partner wish her harm? Of course not. Sometimes the fear that something *could* be wrong results in us making decisions from our minds instead of our bodies, to the detriment of our health.

THE VOICE OF FEAR VS. THE VOICE OF INTUITION

When we've been out of touch with our bodies, it can be difficult to know the difference between the voice of fear and the voice of intuition. The mind-based decisions and the body-based decisions. What I've come to find is this…

Mind-Based Decisions

We know we're using our minds to make decisions when we're finding reasons to validate our decisions. Often, we're taking action because of what we think others will think or how we think it will make us look because we're scared to lose resources like time and money, or we believe we'll get them.

One way to know you're making a decision from your mind is there will often be a conscious reason why you're doing it.

Certainty isn't knowing the answer. It's trusting how you feel.

Body-Based Decisions

Body-based decisions are really what your intuition is. A great way to differentiate between a head decision and a body decision is whether or not you can find a logical reason why you're making a decision. With body-based decisions, it's often a stillness, a knowing, a grounded yes or no. There's often no reason you can give—it's just a yes, or it's a no. It feels calm in the body. Even though it can be a tough decision and you may feel sad about it, you know it's right.

Human beings survived and evolved over millions of years because animals pay attention to their gut feelings. It's not something you have to develop; it's something you have to remember. You already have it. We're just turning the volume up.

When it's your intuition. It's a knowing. Someone can ask you why you made a decision, and you often can't find the words. It's a "it was just the right thing to do" kind of situation. At its core, intuition is that "gut feeling."

Ideally, we use our minds as a resource, like a pros and cons list, and our bodies to make the final decision. We can access all of the information, skills, and tools we've learned across our lifetimes as a mental resource, but, ultimately, we could have a stack of pros and still decide to say no, because the decisions we make are based on our bodies.

I've found that making body-based decisions requires three main things: feeling safe in my body, my ability to connect to my body, and having trust that whatever comes up I can handle.

Let's start with safety.

Finding Safety

I recently had my first colonic, where a lovely woman tried her best to help me relax and feel safe all while flushing gushing water up my bum! Yes, I realize this is A LOT of a story to jump headfirst into, but now you get a glimpse of how unprepared I was too.

You know when you're stressed and someone says, "Just relax."? This was one of those scenarios. The water was pushing up against some gas I had because silly me forgot to prep beforehand, and I love a glass or two of sparkling water. This caused me to feel a mixture of intense abdominal pain, nausea, sweats, and flashbacks of one too many times overseas almost not making it to the toilet with the dreaded "Bali Belly." In this instance, as you can imagine, I didn't want to be in my body. I wanted to be as far away from the situation as possible. I didn't want to feel the pain, the awkwardness, the sensation that I was quite literally going to shit myself on this table in front of the lady with the bum hose. My point is, when we don't feel safe in our bodies, the last thing we want to do is fully feel the emotion. We use humor to aid our experience, or we numb out, disassociate, shut down—go anywhere but where we are.

When we feel scared to be in our bodies...

Sometimes for any number of reasons we can feel like our body is not a safe space to be, and we can feel like if we allow the feelings to fully come, they won't go. So we push them down. *The thing is, we can't selectively push down one emotion, all of them get suppressed.*

Have you ever had an event or birthday that you were going to and beforehand received some bad news? What happens, you go to enjoy yourself, but you just can't seem to get to the same level of enjoyment you normally can. You try to push down the negative feeling about the bad news, but you end up blocking your ability to feel your joyous emotions too.

When we don't have safety, we can't fully feel...

I think of how we process emotions to be like a cup of water. When we inevitably experience things throughout the day, our cup can start to fill up. It's our job to drink that water, to feel the emotions that come from the experiences and allow them to pass through us. The water isn't bad. It gives our bodies the nourishment they need to respond to our inner and outer world. The joy shows us what lights our souls on fire, what we need more of in our lives. The anger shows us that a boundary we hold has been crossed. The jealousy we feel about something shows us what we desire.

When we cling onto the emotion, or shut it down, we don't empty the cup. It keeps getting fuller and fuller and fuller, and all it takes is a little knock for the water to overflow and tip out onto everyone else. We can blame the person who knocked us, or we can become aware of the small amounts of water being added to our cups, and we can drink the water as it's being added, allowing it to pass through us.

Some of you might be thinking, *Those emotions don't feel like water in a cup, they feel like poison! I don't want to drink them. I'm scared they'll make me sicker.* And to that, I say—*Amen.* Our bodies are doing what they think they must to protect us. They're doing what they do best. It can be helpful to use the strategy of not drinking our emotions in moments when they're too much for our bodies. Just like you wouldn't try to drink a glass of water when you're asleep, there's a time and a place to fully feel your emotions—but the water doesn't go away. Unfortunately, you're not made of Gor-Tex; you're more like a sponge.

As someone who used to suppress her emotions, I would often completely miss these subtle messages from my body. I was scared that if I allowed them in, that's what I would feel like forever. What I've learned firsthand is, when we drink the water, it runs out. When we resist and suppress, the water sits there, feeling like it's going to last forever, and it begins to leak out into other parts of our lives.

When we drink the water—feel our emotions close to when we experience them—the water is nourishing to the body, just like drinking a fresh glass of water. Or maybe it's even a glass of day-old or week-old water. Not as nice, but still nourishing to the body. When we suppress and avoid these feelings over a longer period of time, those emotions can become stagnant—but what does this mean?

What Happens When we Don't Process Our Emotions?

When we don't let ourselves process, allowing the water to flow, it builds up and becomes toxic to our bodies. Like a decade-old glass of water.

Four-year-old me, who didn't feel safe to feel her terrified emotions, didn't know how to express herself. She held on to the fear, and that fear leaked out in the form of chronic UTIs. As I got older, the fear leaked out in other ways—crushing chest pain when I didn't speak up and skin breakouts when I continued to allow my boundaries to be crossed.

There are many ancient philosophies and Eastern medicines, such as Chinese medicine, kinesiology, chakra systems, German new medicine, spinal energetics, and many more, that speak to the body keeping score. That's when emotions are too significant to feel at the time and our bodies store them away to be processed later. Unfortunately, a lot of us forget to come back later. Thankfully, Western medicine is starting to acknowledge this too.

Adverse Childhood Experiences (ACE) studies highlight that experiencing significant trauma before the age of 18 increases the risk of developing a chronic illness. The higher your score when assessing risk factors, the more likely you are to develop a chronic illness later in life.[33]

When significant trauma occurs at a young age, we often don't have the tools to know how to process it. Like not knowing how to drink from a sippy cup when we're a toddler. When we don't process the event, our bodies hold on to it as a form of protection, to remember. This is a survival mechanism. It's beneficial, until it becomes toxic to your body, like drinking a 10-year-old glass of water.

We're often conditioned to resist, reject, and hate the parts of our bodies we want to change. If you're experiencing any kind of physical body symptoms—for example, PCOS, acne, painful periods, IBS, depression, anxiety, fluid retention—it could be a sign that you're not making decisions from your body.

Bodily Issues and Interlinked Energetics

Different tissues in our bodies seem to be affected by holding on to certain emotions. If you experience chronic issues with a part of your body, consider looking at the energetics of this tissue.

Menstrual cycle

Where are you invalidating yourself, not trusting your intuition, and instead using fear to guide you? Our intuition is a cornerstone of our femininity. You may feel more compelled by fear and lack of control than trust and intuition. What's your relationship to experiencing sensuality and pleasure?

A 2018 study found that there was a correlation between women who had experienced physical or sexual abuse in early life and the development of endometriosis, with a 79 percent increased risk of developing endometriosis if the incidence was severe or repeated.[34]

Gut

Where are you finding trouble with letting go of past hurts, or holding on to grudges? We can struggle with procrastination and not knowing how to move forward, often seeing others as the problem and being inclined to act like a victim.

What thought, belief, or pattern of behavior do you need to let go of?

Sleep

Where in your life are you feeling unsafe, threatened, helpless, vulnerable, or on guard? When we experience sleep troubles, it can be that our bodies deem it unsafe to have time for resetting, or you're under perceived threat now. What is your relationship to rest and relaxation?

Energy

Where in your life are you over-giving? Experiencing energy troubles can mean you have an imbalance between giving and receiving. Notice your energy around giving. Are you expecting something in return? Do you find it hard to receive? This could be in the form of compliments, attention, support, or money.

Hair

Hair acts as insulation for your head and your body. It also helps to produce natural self-cleaning and protective oils. If you're experiencing issues with your hair, ask yourself, *Where am I noticing anger, guilt, frustration, resentment, or sadness?*

Skin

What is your relationship to anger? Anger is a gift letting us know a boundary has been crossed. Our skin is the physical boundary between us and the world. It's flexible and responsive to change but still resilient. Where are you allowing others, or yourself, to cross a boundary you've set? Do you know what your boundaries are? Have you communicated them?

Nails

Where in your life are you feeling frustrated? Is there something or someone that's hanging around like a hangnail? Do you think something is taking too long? What small frustrations can you delegate or remove in your life?

Tongue and mouth

Cat got your tongue? Often, tongue issues are associated with not saying what you need to say because of fear. What are you not saying? What old hurts are you holding on to?

Vulva

Are you putting others before yourself, falling into the mothering role for others in your life? What is your reaction to being called selfish? What do you need? You need to balance the giving and receiving. Ask for what you need, or give it to yourself. Are you holding on to past hurts, shame, or humiliation?

Uterus

Where in your life do you lack certainty or clarity? Are you supporting yourself or asking for support from others when you need it? Where are you living your life for yourself? Where are you living your life for the approval of others? Offer yourself more appreciation and compassion.

Breasts

What are you doing that you don't want to be doing? Where are you giving others support and don't believe you also deserve the same?

The breast is a nurturing organ. Often, issues with the breast can arise when you don't accept or give yourself nourishment and support.

Immune system

Where in your life do you need to say no? Where have you over-loaded yourself? Do you know what your boundaries are? Have you communicated them? Are you ignoring the signals of your body and allowing your to-do list or others' expectations to run your life? Where are you neglecting your true wants and desires for the benefit of the outside world?

Find the balance between what's best for you and what's best for the collective.

Did you know that 80 percent of people who experience auto-immune disorders are women?[35] Autoimmune disorders occur when our bodies confuse self for others. When we forgo and minimize the needs of self for the needs of others on a regular basis, we can lose connection with what "self" even looks like. Interestingly, this is the fawn response. Although there's no evidence to suggest a physiological difference in brain matter among males and females, it seems women are more socialized to believe fawning and keeping the happiness of everyone else is important for the happiness and safety of themselves, whereas men aren't as affected by this.

Signs you don't feel safe to feel

Freeze/fawn response to avoid feelings and find protection:
- "Cool girl"—nothing really phases you
- Ghosting people
- Binge eating or drinking
- Drug use

- Alcohol
- Social media addiction
- People-pleasing
- Disassociating
- Not being able to communicate how you feel (knowing something is off but not knowing what)
- Not asking for help
- Always deflecting to humor
- High pain threshold
- Ruminating over the same thoughts over and over

Fight/flight response to avoid feelings and find protection:
- Trouble sitting still
- Low pain threshold
- Finding it difficult to be in silence
- Highly reactive
- Conflict avoidant
- Conflict seeking—looking to others to feel your pain
- Feeling like you're in a rush… Think about this—it's literally resisting where you are right now, thinking you should be somewhere else. You walk fast, talk fast, drive fast. Everything has to be done yesterday.

Just like drinking a glass of water on the toilet probably isn't recommended, most of us would prefer not to release ten years'

worth of trauma on our long-lost friend in aisle seven of the supermarket. There's a time and a place. That time and place is where we feel safe.

If you find that you have a particularly high aversion to feeling your feelings, have a history of addiction, or experience many of the above, I recommend finding a practitioner you trust who can guide you on the journey of finding safety in your body.

If you feel like you can cultivate a level of safety in your environment yourself and have an existing support network around you, in the next section, you'll learn how to get started with connecting to your body.

When I say you don't feel safe, this doesn't mean you never feel safe. We can move in and out of safety throughout the day. Sometimes, however, we haven't felt enough safety to hold the bigger, older glasses of water.

CONNECTION TO BODY

In order to make decisions from our bodies, we must first be able to connect to them.

Some signs you're not connected to your body

- Diagnosed with a chronic illness
- Period pain
- Binge eating or drinking
- Addictive tendencies
- Inability to sit still
- Saying yes to things when you really want to say no

Things that can take you out of connection with your body

- Thinking about the future
- Thinking about the past
- Alcohol
- Medication
- Pornography
- Illicit drugs
- Chronic thinking about others' needs
- Lack of movement
- Significant trauma (psychosocial or physical)
- Scrolling social media
- Saying yes when you really want to say no

How we can become disconnected

- The body perceives it's unsafe to feel. What it was experiencing was too much to hold at the time, so dissociation was the best response (a healthy response to an abnormal environment).
- Choosing not to act on the subtle signs from the body (such as not going to the toilet when you need to).
- Ignoring your own wants and desires. It could be something as simple as a takeaway night with your friends, where you just go along with what others want when you really don't want to.
- Accepting certain treatment for a condition when you don't want to.
- Medications like pain killers and hormonal contraceptives, which mask body signs.

CONNECTING TO EMOTIONS

I used to struggle with feeling and understanding my emotions. I was someone who would push them down, not realizing what I was doing. I'd always feel pretty good, never amazing but also never usually terrible. On occasion, my mum would ask me how I was feeling or what was going on, and I literally couldn't find the words to describe how I was feeling. I knew something was off, but I had no idea what, or how I could explain it. There was nothing. This is a common way of feeling when you struggle to connect with your body and how you feel.

There's a reason why we often interchange the words emotions and feelings. Emotions are meant to be felt. They're generated from a certain frequency of vibration that our cells create. David R. Hawkins called this the scale of consciousness.[36] This vibration can change the amount of heat, turbulence, and movement that's generated, hence why your body feels different when you're angry than when you're jumping for joy.

In fact, a 2011 study found that emotional states have distinct sensations in the body, and these are universal across cultures and life events.[37] Essentially, how certain emotions, like anger, surprise, love, and anxiety, feel in my body are the same as how they feel in your body. When we feel heat and energy in the upper chest and arms, we're feeling angry. When we feel a calm heat all over the body, radiating from the chest, we're feeling happy.

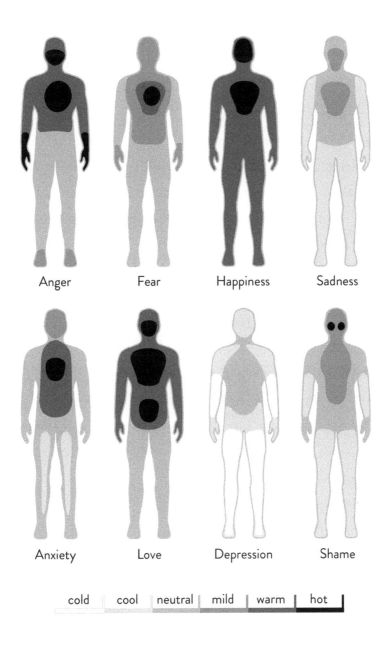

Emotional changes help to alter our physiology so we can survive the challenges present in our environments, adjusting our hormones, cardiovascular system, muscle activation, and automatic functions. We don't think about making our hands sweaty and rapidly pounding our heart before giving a big speech. It can just happen.

The catch is, it depends on the context in which we feel these emotions. For instance, you might feel a rush of sensation through your torso and into your limbs as a result of a surprise party and feel a sense of excitement, or you might feel that same rush when you hear a gunshot and experience fear. Both the physical sensation and the context matters.

Feelings and emotions are subtle signs the body is telling you something.

The same goes for when we suppress, ignore, or avoid our emotions. When we hold on to the water in our cups and let it sit there for days, weeks, and years on end, we miss the gift. We miss the signal from the body that's trying to keep us on track. When we don't find time for it, or we don't have safety to feel, it can eventually boil over, typically, in reactive behaviors or, worse, in the form of disease.

Emotions can be triggered from an external stimulus, for example, someone crossing one of your boundaries, resulting in anger. Or they can also be triggered from an internal stimulus, for example, having high amounts of cortisol in your body, adding caffeine to the mix, and having a bowl of cereal for breakfast. This combination of cortisol and insulin creates high blood sugar, triggering a higher resting heart rate and a feeling of anxiety.[38]

Option	External trigger	Internal resources	Outcome
A	Someone cuts you off in traffic	You're well-rested and fed	Slightly annoyed and forget about it
B	Someone cuts you off in traffic	You're exhausted, depleted, and hungry	Road rage, anger

The output we experience is a combination of what we're exposed to externally and the internal environment, or raw materials, of our systems.

So, should you trust your emotions? Yes. Are they always coming from the place you think they are? Possibly not.

CONNECTING TO YOUR EMOTIONS

"Emotions are energy in motion."

Emotions offer a gift from the body letting us know something, so when we don't allow ourselves to feel our anger, sadness, joy, or happiness, we miss the gift. We miss the subtle messages from our bodies.

Anxiety

Occurs when something or someone has the potential to be harmful. If we didn't have anxiety, we wouldn't survive, as it provides safety and awareness. However, when it's dialed way up, it can prevent us from living joyful lives by being in the present moment.

Anger

Highlights that a boundary we hold has been crossed. Either we've crossed it ourselves, or someone else has crossed it.

Contempt

Shows us our values, what we wish for other people, and where we can soften and approach from curiosity instead of judgment.

Depression

Could be showing us that the body lacks adequate nourishment and raw materials or that it wants us to change something in our lives, for example, our environment.

Disgust

Shows us what is absolutely not for us, something we want to move far away from.

Disappointment

A sign that we may need to communicate our expectations more clearly or that others aren't fulfilling them.

Envy

Shows us what we want by seeing it in others.

Excitement

Shows us something we want more of, the direction we need to move.

Fear

The gift of protecting us from perceived danger and death.

Happiness

The gift of feeling safe.

Love

The gift of connection to others.

Neutral

The gift of balance. When we don't feel it, we know there's an imbalance.

Pride

The gift of feeling good about ourselves.

Resentment

We need to set boundaries for ourselves and ask for more of what we need.

Sadness

Shows us what we value through what we might lose.

Shame

Indicates that the action we've taken is misaligned with the picture we have of ourselves.

Surprise

The gift of uncertainty.

～

Still not sold on your emotions working in your favor? Think of it this way—when we, for example, cut ourselves, the pain and the bleeding are a gift. A gift to show us how we need to tend to our wounds. There are people in this world who can't detect pain; they have a condition called congenital insensitivity to pain and anhidrosis (CIPA). It's extremely rare, and they have a high risk of early death because they can't detect the things that are causing damage to their bodies. Touching a hot stove, jumping from a height and breaking an ankle, developing pressure sores because they haven't moved in bed. A similar thing happens when diabetics start to lose sensation in their limbs. They can have ulcers that go unfelt and if the area isn't checked regularly, these ulcers can turn septic, leading to possible full-body infection and, in some cases, death.

When you're attuned to your emotions, you understand that they're all important and are telling you something. So, when you dive deep, listen inside, and feel the tears of sadness, of happiness, of overwhelm start to come, allow them to flow—*the water feeds your growth*. When you dive inside and feel the heat start to come, allow it to burn, to smoke out what doesn't belong in your life—*to clear a new path forward*. When you dive inside and feel the turbulence start to build, allow it to come and shake what needs to be let go of—*and allow what needs to stay, stay.*

HOW DO WE START TO FEEL OUR EMOTIONS?

Like watching a toddler learn how to drink from a cup for the first time, when we haven't learned how to feel our emotions, it can feel like we're being waterboarded. It can feel all too much too soon, and out of our control. The first step in learning to drink the water is to find safety in our bodies and environments.

When we find it difficult to feel safe in our own bodies, or we lack safety in our physical and emotional relationships, our bodies resist fully feeling the emotions as a way to protect us. It's precisely the reason why we didn't feel them in the first place. We shut down, numb, or run away from the emotion, leaving us feeling reactive and unsettled. This is a healthy response in the beginning, but, as we've covered, it becomes unhealthy the longer we allow it to go on.

How to Connect to Your Body

There are hundreds of different exercises, modalities, and medicines that can help you connect with your body. Your body is a physical thing, so the easiest way to connect to it is to connect to the feeling and different somatic sensations.

These are some of my personal favorites

- **Start your day with ten deep breaths**. With each breath in and out, connect to a different body part and come from the point of view of breathing from that part. For instance, breath one, I'm breathing in from my heart and out from my heart; breath two, I'm breathing in from my liver and out from my liver; breath three, in and out from my uterus, and so on. You can literally use the body from your earlobe to your big toe.

- **Play**. Do things for the sake of it. Jump in the pool with your clothes on, do a cartwheel, do the things you used to do as a kid.

- **Pleasure**. This could be a warm bath, self-pleasure practice, massage, listening to your favorite song, or eating your favorite food.

- **Put on a love song,** and, as you're singing along, imagine the words are coming from a part of your body and directed at you (for example, play Whitney Houston's "I Will Always Love You").

- **Connect to your mmmmhhh**. After being in my body, what I've come to realize is that I uncontrollably find myself saying "mmmmhhh" throughout the day. Look at a sunset? "Mmmmhhh." Look at a sunrise? "Mmmmhhh." Feel the sensation of clean bed sheets? "Mmmmhhh." Hear a group of people laughing? "Mmmmhhh." Look at a picture of Ryan Reynolds… You get the picture. The sound of mmmmhhh actually works to stimulate your vagus nerve with the contraction of specific palate muscles. The vagus nerve is responsible for the calming effects on the internal body, the green lights, effectively giving a hug and a word of encouragement to all of your internal organs.

- **Do what your body's basic functions are telling you**. Cold? Put on a jumper. Need to go to the toilet? Go to the toilet. Don't like the way your clothes feel? Get changed. Tolerance for discomfort is a helpful skill but when we normalize it, we can normalize disconnecting from our bodies.
- **Conscious movement**. Consciously paying attention to your body through different movements will help you to connect to it, for example, doing different yoga poses and sending your attention to different body parts.

These practices may seem small and unimportant to you, but they build the muscle between messages from your body and you taking action. When this connection is strong, our lives can be based on what's best for our bodies.

Simple Embodiment Exercise

1. Feel safe in your body by connecting to your "green lights" that we refer to in Chapter 4. This includes a safe environment as well as connecting to one of what Richard Swartz terms the 8Cs: calm, curiosity, creativity, compassion, clarity, confidence, courage, or connectedness. I personally find that being curious about what my body might tell me and having compassion for my body helps me connect deeper.
2. Connect to your breath as a window into your body and scan around your body for any sensations that

start to arise. They could be heat, tension, numbness, turbulence, cold, dullness, and so on (there's no right or wrong here).

3. If you find that nothing is coming to you, or that you're finding it difficult to drop into your body, try imagining each breath in and out coming from a different organ of your body. Breathing in and out from your liver, from your skin, from your heart, your eyes, your toes, and so on.

4. You may then start to notice some physical sensations in your body. This is your body showing you where that "water" is being stored.

5. This is gut instinct. Go with the first thing that comes up. When we first start to do this, sometimes we can override and second-guess with our minds. That's OK—go with what first comes up.

6. Notice the sensation with a gentle curiosity and sit with it, allowing it to soften. You can even ask your body, *Is there anything you'd like to let me know?*

7. Allow your body to move in whatever way it feels like moving. You may want to shake, cry, laugh, cough, twist, wreath around, or be still. Keep breathing and allow the sensation to move, shift, and change in your body.

8. You may notice that the sensation starts to change or dissipate.

9. You've just taken a drink of some of the water.

Good Morning Routine

You can incorporate several of these into a morning routine, waking up to some conscious body part breathing and asking your body: *What, if anything, do you need? What would be the best way to start the day for you?* This could lead to a nice self-massage, some more conscious breathing, or even a naked dance party to your favorite song in your bedroom. The key is to ask your body. Just because you booked in that early morning workout class doesn't mean you're a lazy piece of shit for not going. Sometimes the best thing for our bodies is listening to what they actually need. *But sometimes that workout class is exactly what your body needs.*

You'll find more tools and resources for supporting your energetic health on our website and via the links in the Resources section at the back of the book.

Signs you are connected to your body

- Noticing sensation in the body before consciously realizing what it is.
- Noticing you're making more decisions based on how you feel compared to what you *think* you should be doing.
- You're in the driver's seat. You've developed a relative sense of control of your life.

~

If you've noticed that you may be holding on to some past hurts that are affecting your body and your life, and you don't quite know how to feel or process the feelings, and you want to care for your energetic health as well, you can support yourself by connecting to your body every day and asking it with tender curiosity:

- "Is there anything you'd like to let me know?"
- "Do you have any information you'd like to share with me?"
- "Is there any important information you feel I should be aware of?"
- "Would you like to share anything with me?"
- "Is there something you want to let me in on?"
- "Do you have any messages or updates for me?"
- "Is there anything you'd like to bring to my attention?"
- "Is there something you think I should know about?"

First, we find safety.
Second, we connect and feel.
Third, we trust ourselves.

Trust What Comes Up

Many of us have been conditioned to distrust the feelings of our bodies, over time, being told we're too sensitive so we're the problem, or that the emotions are too much—the emotions are the problem. When this happens, our bodies start to become deaf to the sensations because they think that's best for survival. Our bodies always want survival. So, if this is you, thank your body. It's been doing everything necessary to get you here.

I often think about this when I'm sitting with my emotions and they're really not fun to feel. Let's face it, most of us don't automatically jump for joy and think, *I want to feel stressed, bored, sad, angry all the time. I love this feeling!*

What I've come to realize from knowing that my body has my best interests at heart is that when the sensation arises, it's bringing the feeling to the surface because **I am meant to feel it.** (Feeling doesn't mean acting on).

I imagine it like being at a family party, in a room full of adults, and one of the toddlers is running around trying to find someone to console them because they grazed their knee. Or they're looking for someone to jump for joy with them because they found a new toy. When they choose you to show you, it means they feel safe with you, safe to express these feelings. Whether it's happiness, sadness, anger, frustration, guilt, shame, it's a privilege to feel it. It feels safe to come to the surface, just like the toddler does when they choose an adult to experience an emotion with.

When the toddler is acknowledged, often the tears or the joy last only momentarily. The same is true for our emotions. Dr. Jill Bolte Taylor writes about the 90-second cycle of emotion: "There's a 90-second chemical process that happens in the body; after that, any remaining emotional response is just the person choosing to stay in that emotional loop."[39] What she means is that it's our thoughts that keep that physiological cycle of discomfort running on a loop. Sometimes the "choice" to stay in the loop is our resistance to the feeling. I often see this with patients who don't want to cry.

**"Crying is the best, isn't it?
It's like an orgasm for the soul."
—Rebecca (*Ted Lasso*)**

Before I developed the skill of feeling the emotion fully, I would find that the sensation would come and then it would sort of hang around, never quite reaching climax. Now, when the wave of emotion is fully felt, the post-crying orgasm for the soul is a real thing! Who are you to deny your soul an orgasm?

When we don't trust ourselves and our own realities...

In recent years, it has become more common to talk about medical gaslighting. For those of you who are unaware, gaslighting refers to someone questioning their own reality. In blatant terms, it's when you see your sister borrow your T-shirt and you ask her if she did, and she denies it so much that it makes you question whether you saw her take it in the first place. In healthcare, it's when you feel like there's something wrong with your body and you're convinced by others that everything is fine, that it's "in your head."

When we don't trust how we feel, or we're constantly putting the needs of others before our own and denying our own realities, we're more susceptible to gaslighting, and we can end up gaslighting ourselves.

This is what happened to me when the flashbacks of being 4 years old, feeling terrified and sexually abused, started. I would convince myself that they were random intrusive thoughts, that everyone must have them, and I would push them down and move on with my day, gaslighting myself into believing there was no way anything like that could have happened to me. The more they came, the more I wanted to deny my reality, convincing myself that it was better to think I was making it up than it was to know that it was true. Thanks to the amazing support of numerous practitioners, my friends, and my family, I began to trust myself. Now, when I notice small instances of denying my personal reality, coming back to my body and listening to what it's telling me helps ground me.

The safety to sit with your emotions and then trust them is one of the most life-changing things you'll ever develop.

Support and Guidance From Others

If you're someone who feels "dead below the neck," spends a lot of time in their mind, or finds they deny their own reality a lot of the time, I recommend seeking guidance from a practitioner who can help you connect to your body.

Body-based practitioners

- Kinesiology
- Spinal energetics
- Reiki
- Somatic-based workers, like massage therapists, chiropractors and more…
- PARTS work

Brain-based practitioners

- Psychology
- Cognitive behavioral therapy
- Acceptance and commitment therapy (ACT)
- PARTS work

~~

As you become more attuned to your body, you'll often start to notice the subtle bodily sensations before you consciously recognize the emotions you're feeling, meaning you can feel the heat in your hands and face before you consciously realize you're angry.

When we connect to our bodies and find safety in them, it builds foundations of trust in ourselves. That trust can be lifesaving, like in the instance of my patient, Sandra, with the abdominal tumor, and it can also improve the quality of your life.

Remember, our emotions, like the water in our glasses, are good for us. I'd much rather drink a cup of fresh water than a cup of water that has been sitting there for days, weeks, years, or even decades. The longer the water sits there, the more likely it is to cause disease. The water doesn't sit separately to us; it sits in us, unless we allow it to move through us, giving us the nourishment and guidance we need.

This doesn't mean you have to scull the water as soon as it enters your glass. Think of it like hydrating, sipping the water across the day. We can allow the water to sit there for some time and slowly pick it up to drink when we need it. The key is to not let it sit there for too long.

Some questions that can be helpful to ask about your body

- Does it feel like my energy is coming from within or from outside sources?
- What is my body craving right now?
- What would be nourishing to my body?
- What am I doing daily that is keeping me in this pattern?
- If I could let go of one belief about myself, what would that be?
- If my dearest friend was feeling how I am, what would I feel they need?

Remember, emotions are your reality. They're valid, yes—we need to feel in order to heal. *And* we can take what we need from them and know that our emotions are not us. They don't make us inherently one way or another. Because we experience anxiety, it doesn't mean we'll always be anxious. The anxiety is the output. It's a symptom. It's the feedback from the body, letting us know how our internal, raw-material body is responding to the external environment we're putting it in.

Just like with a rash or a broken arm, the feeling is important. It shows you what you need to see, but it isn't you.

> **"What you are is what you have been.**
> **What you'll be is what you do now."**
> **—Buddha**

TIME FOR A NEW REALITY

I recommend grabbing a pen and journal to answer some of these questions for yourself.

A couple of weeks ago, someone asked me if I could go and buy them something from the shops. It was something I had never bought before. A lottery ticket. My brain was literally thinking, *How do I even buy one of these? Where's the store? I've never seen it before.* I had to ask someone else where the store was. You'll never guess—it was right beside the entrance to the supermarket I go to multiple times a week. Yet I hadn't registered that it was there. My eyes would have seen it, yet nothing. It didn't register in my mind. Why?

The answer lies in the concept that while we're all living at the same point in time, maybe the exact same moment in time, we're all experiencing a different reality. So, there isn't one reality, but rather over 8 billion realities occurring at one time. The reason why lies in the stories we are consistently telling ourselves. The best part is, the story you most believe will always win.

A famous example of this is the 2011 "Mind over Milkshakes" research study. In the study, researchers divided the sample of participants into two groups and served them all the same milkshake. One group was told the milkshake was high in calories, sugar, and fat. The other group was told it was low in calories, sugar, and fat. Again, they all had the exact same milkshake. The result… Those who were told they had consumed the higher-calorie, sugary, fatty (bad) milkshake experienced a "steeper decline" in the hunger hormone ghrelin than those in the low-calorie, low-sugar, low-fat (good) group, who didn't experience the same level of ghrelin decline, therefore, didn't feel as satiated.[40]

So, what happened?

Those who were told it was a high-calorie, high-sugar, high-fat milkshake believed they were consuming a large number of calories, creating both a mental and physical feeling of satiation. Those who believed they were drinking a "healthy" milkshake thought they were getting fewer calories, and their bodies seemingly went along with it, refusing to significantly lower their hunger hormones. It had nothing to do with the food itself.

**It's the stories we believe about ourselves
that create our reality.**

I believe I'm not a gambler, so I didn't see the lottery ticket store. The study participants believed the milkshake was healthy or unhealthy, and their bodies responded differently. Whether or not a story is true or not doesn't matter to our bodies; it's what we believe that matters.

**"Whether you think you can,
or you think you can't—you're right."
—Henry Ford**

Placebo is another classic example of how our beliefs and expectations can alter our results. Placebo is the thought that something will give us a positive response. For example, commonly in randomized control trials, an active drug, say Viagra, and an inactive drug, a sugar pill, are given without telling the participants which pill they received. Researchers randomize who gets which drug and take note of who gets the desired outcome, in the case of Viagra, an erection. If there is a high percentage of men who get an erection after taking the placebo pill compared to taking the active pill, or the percentages are similar, then the placebo effect is high. Basically, the placebo effect demonstrates that for certain subjects, their belief about what they were taking (thinking it was an active ingredient) would give them the same result as the actual active substance, even when no active substance was present.

Just as we have the placebo effect, we can also have the nocebo effect. This can occur when we have negative expectations or beliefs regarding the outcome of a treatment. So, in other words, if you expect the outcome of something to be bad, you're more likely to experience a bad response. This effect has been demonstrated in studies where side effects of drugs have been highlighted to patients before they take them.[41]

Both the placebo and nocebo effect highlight the power of the mind, expectations, and the importance of choosing which beliefs we pour our energy into.

THE DIAGNOSIS ISN'T THE DESTINATION

I think about all of the women who suffer with debilitating period pain, heavy periods, changes with their bowels with their menstrual cycles, painful sex, and sometimes trouble with their fertility, thinking they're going crazy… until the third, fourth, tenth time they visit a doctor, and they're finally told, "We know what's wrong. You have endometriosis." A feeling of relief comes when they realize they aren't crazy and there is actually something wrong. This can be life-changing in and of itself—the act of being seen. However, the relief can be momentary because the diagnosis sets up a belief that alters their reality.

Be careful what your diagnosis is making you believe

Our beliefs program the destinations of our GPSs. Whether we realize it or not, we have been contributing to the destination of our health. The consistency in the stories we tell ourselves are creating highways in our bodies. It's like when you drive the same route from home to work—you arrive and think to yourself, *Did I go straight through that red light? What about that stop sign?* The pattern and drive are so ingrained in our neural pathways that our bodies make a lot of the actions subconscious to conserve energy, and we end up never questioning them because they're so automatic. When we do things on autopilot, these neural pathways are like well-worn tracks that get us to where we want to go with minimal effort.

Remember, your beliefs shape your journey, and a diagnosis can shape your beliefs.

Essentially, a diagnosis is a label that helps others understand what you could be feeling or experiencing. However, how the healthcare system views your condition doesn't provide you with any more answers as to why you're experiencing it in the first place.

Instead of believing that your diagnosis means there's something wrong with you, it can be much more beneficial to believe it's a sign that your body is working for you. It's showing you exactly what you need to see. It's just that now someone has put a label on what it has been showing you all along.

So, What are the Stories You Believe About Yourself?

Common stories I hear from patients are:

- "My mum had endometriosis, so I'm probably going to have it too."
- "I always get period pain, and I probably always will."
- "I feel like crap because I'm getting old" (said a 29-year-old, 35-year-old, 47-year-old, 63-year-old, and an 85-year-old…). *Hint—We're always getting older; it doesn't mean you have to feel crap.*
- "Every new mum feels like this, it's normal."
- "You'll have fun with me, no one can figure out what's wrong."
- "Are you ready? I'm really complex, I've got so many issues going on."

Common stories you might be telling yourself that can be affecting your health

- *Gut problems are normal for me.*
- *I'm just a little bit broken.*
- *That's just the way my body was made.*
- *I don't have time.*
- *Depression runs in my family.*
- *Diabetes runs in the family, so…*
- *It's out of my control.*
- *Person X brings out the worst in me.*
- *You're not meant to enjoy your work.*
- *I've always been a night owl.*
- *To celebrate, you have to have (insert substance).*
- *When you go out, you have to have alcohol.*
- *Crying means you're weak.*
- *If I say how I feel, people will leave me.*
- *I'm quite an anxious person.*
- *If I don't go to the gym every day, then I'll be fat and lazy.*

You might notice some resistance come up when you read these.

"Well, gut problems are normal for me!"

"My mum did have endometriosis!"

"I do always get period pain!"

"I am actually really complex!"

If you're noticing any resistance coming up when your beliefs are challenged, this is good. Becoming aware is the first step. Now become curious…

Pull out your journal now and get curious about the stories you believe about yourself.

Are You Getting a Kink out of Your Current Reality?

Sometimes we say we want to change our reality, but the benefits of what we're getting from the current situation are too great for us to want to change.

In early high school, when my heart condition and surgeries were happening, I would play what I used to call the "heart card" when I didn't want to do something at school. Why not use it to my advantage, right?

I'm a lover of sport, and competition is fun for me, but I loathed the beep test and cross-country. So, when it would come time to do the yearly beep test—heart card. There couldn't possibly be a way that I could do the beep test. Same with cross country. But could I play a full day of round-robin soccer matches in 30°C (86°F) heat? Basketball matches? Netball? One-hundred-meter sprints? Yes, of course I could do all that—because I enjoyed those activities. If I had chest pain before or even throughout, I would still keep playing. (If any of my high school PE teachers are reading this, yes, I was lying, whoops!). Often, my nails would turn blue, and sometimes I'd need the next day off of school because of how exhausted I was (I don't recommend trying this at home). But the key here is that in some way, I was getting a kink out of my belief about my heart.

If you want to dive deeper into this, *Existential Kink* by Carolyn Elliot is a must-read.

What are the benefits of your stories?

When you look at the stories you're repeating in your life, what possible benefit could you be getting from them?

Below are some examples from some of my patients:

- You might want to get out of going to school or to a birthday dinner for Susan down the road, so your migraines play up.
- You might have seen your parents work really hard and then get sick, so you believe you can't have a great job, work hard, and be healthy, so you avoid making an effort.
- Being sick gives you love and attention from others, so you get sick more often.
- You hate school, and period pain gives you a day off.
- Diagnosis and frequent symptoms provide "proof" of the story "my body is broken."

Get curious about how your current life could be benefiting you and write this in your journal.

Ultimately, it's you who gets to decide which stories you tell yourself and which you reject. It's you who decides how to interpret the messages of your body. It's you who gets to program your GPS.

You could have the story of

- "I'm too busy to go to the gym, I'll go when I've finished this big project."
- "That's not how my parents did it."
- "It's too difficult to start a new job."
- "Everyone feels like this at my age."
- "I'm always the one who gets sick."
- "Why me?"
- "It's normal to feel like this."
- "Being overweight runs in my family."
- "Three generations of my family died of heart disease, so I'll probably die of it too."
- "My mum had endometriosis, so that's probably why I have painful periods."
- "All my grandparents lived to over one hundred, so I'll be around for quite a while."
- "Mental illness runs in our family, we're all just anxious."
- "Everyone in my family is overweight, so of course I am too. *We don't run in our jeans.*"
- "The doctor said I had to come back and get tested next year to see if I might need medication then."

You might also have the story of

- "My body is responding exactly how it needs to."
- "My body is always supporting me."
- "I can do whatever I set my mind to."

- "Why not me?"
- "Anything is possible."
- "It's turning out better than I could have imagined."

The most powerful story always wins.

When you subscribe to a particular story, you shape everything else around it to confirm the story to be true. In order to get from where you are to where you want to go, you must first confront whatever is stopping you: the feelings, thoughts, beliefs, and, ultimately, your actions created by your story...

In your journal, word vomit all of the current thoughts, beliefs, roles, actions, feelings, and behaviors that make up who you are now. Title it whatever you wish, for example, past me, old me, something like that.

BUT WHAT ABOUT GENETICS?

I see a lot of patients who often say something along the lines of, "Oh, my mum and my sisters have this, so I probably will too." While, yes, there is a genetic component to a lot of diseases, science is discovering that the role genetics play in the expression of disease is much smaller than we thought, and, really, environment is often what triggers the gene to be expressed or not.[42]

The genes provide the hardware, but how we use it can yield a totally different result, kind of like how you and I both have smartphones. They could be different brands, but we use them to perform similar tasks. You might be more of a texter and I a caller, so the main functions of the phones change. We might even have identical phones, like identical twins, but the way we use them changes how they function. In numerous twin studies, they've shown that our genes aren't our destinations. It's how we use them that matters.

DNA can give you an indication of what *might* happen, but it doesn't tell you what *will* happen. For most chronic illnesses, like PCOS, endometriosis, cancer, type 2 diabetes, and autoimmune disease, lifestyle is a predictive factor. In fact, some research from Dr. Joe Dispenza's work finds that just having different intentions and emotions can signal a gene to make different proteins and promote different actions from cells.[43]

What does all of this mean? Be intentional with what you want and where you want your GPS set.

THE COOLEST THING...

Do you want to know the coolest of cool things about your body? It's *always* adapting. Even if you think you're the most resistant-to-change person ever, I've got news for you: your body has been adapting to create that exact reality. We have no say in whether it does or doesn't change. What we do have a say in is *how* it adapts.

The how is directly correlated with the perceived balance of internal resources for external demands. This influences our epigenetics. So, if you consistently do one thing and it works, your body will learn that pattern, and it will become ingrained. Take, for instance, if you go to the gym consistently, your body shape, fitness, mental state, and physiology as a whole will adapt. If you sit on the couch watching TV all day every day, your body shape and internal physiology will adapt in a completely different way. Like I said, your body is *always* adapting. It's a mirror. So, when we don't like what the mirror is reflecting back, we can look at the story we're telling ourselves that alters our behavior, our internal resources, and our external environment.

What are you focusing on? What do you think is possible for your life? We create this invisible container called our reality, yet this reality is very different from person to person. A group of people could receive the exact same stimulus and have different outputs. Why? Because their internal GPSs are set differently. They make things mean different things. Does that mean that one way is better than another? Or more true than another? I don't think so. But what it does mean is that if you don't like the reality you're currently experiencing, you can change it by changing your perception. How do you do that? You look at your expectations and physiology. You get curious and conscious of the functions that are already self-driving. You become conscious and in charge of where your GPS is set.

THE NEW YOU!

Want to know how your health is going to end up? Ask yourself this simple question… *Where do I think my health is going?*

Although the question is simple, we often don't consciously consider it, yet we do often hold unconscious beliefs that end up leaking into our language and creating the end result we're already geared towards.

"I want to be healthy, fit, and have energy" versus "I don't want to feel tired, fat, and unhealthy anymore." See the difference? It's about designing and creating the life you do want, as opposed to avoiding the one you don't.

Whether you like it or not, you're the creator of your story. It's already unfolding, so you might as well take control now.

The first step when you're beginning to acknowledge the power you have to create your reality is to connect to what Richard Schwartz, the founder of Internal Family Systems, terms the 8 C's, which I mentioned earlier.[44] To jog your memory, the 8 C's are: compassion, curiosity, clarity, creativity, calm, confidence, courage, and connectedness.

When we connect to these 8 C's, we're connecting to our true self energy, giving us a healthy perspective on our patterns and the ability to more readily create change. For example, you might wake up feeling depressed. When we learn that we're creating this reality, it can be a really hard pill to swallow, especially when we're already in a state of depression. How the hell are we meant to figure out how to change our reality when we don't even want to get out of bed in the morning? When we connect to one of the 8 C's, it can help alter our internal dialogue. Here's an example.

Judgment: "Well, clearly I'm just a piece of shit. If I created this feeling, then it must all be my fault."

Curiosity: "I wonder what might be contributing to this feeling I'm experiencing?"

See the difference?

When we remove ourselves from *being* our feelings to *observing* and being *curious* about our feelings, it helps us gain perspective. When we have this perspective, we can see how this is just another way our bodies are talking to us.

Understanding the New You

Word vomit in your journal all your new thoughts, beliefs, roles, actions, feelings, and behaviors that make up who you are now. Name this version of you "The Real (insert name)," "Amazing (insert name)," "(Insert name) 2.0,"… a title that gives you the same goosebumps you feel when something amazing happens.

As you bring the new you into existence, ask yourself these questions:

- What new stories does version 2.0 of you believe?
- What are you feeling?
- What do you believe about yourself?
- What do you believe about others?
- What do people say about you?
- What do you say to yourself?
- What do you do for fun?

- How does your body feel?
- Who are you?

If you're noticing that it's difficult to connect to new beliefs, you'll find tons of helpful resources, like hypnosis and PARTS work in our female fundamentals membership, on our website.

HOW DO YOU CREATE THE LIFE AND HEALTH YOU WANT?

Now that you better understand the new you, it's time to reiterate some of the critical components of creating the life and health you want. Each one is super important, so don't hesitate to revisit this page—or any part of the book—if you ever find yourself feeling lost. Sometimes a little refresher is all it takes to put us back on track.

1. Connect to your body

The best way to keep you on track is to connect to your body, paying attention to the little whispers. This is where your intuition comes from. You feel grounded, and your nervous system regulates.

2. Trust in your body

Remember, your body always has your best interests at heart. If you're experiencing symptoms you don't like, they're not a sign that you're broken; they're showing you what you need to change.

3. Trust in yourself

You can take different actions every day. When you trust yourself, you put yourself in the driver's seat. Trust yourself and know that you are not your beliefs.

4. Know where you want to go

Do an inventory of all the stories you're telling yourself about yourself. The good and the bad. Sit down and curiously see the benefits you're getting from these stories. Know that this is where your GPS is currently programmed. Connect to the knowing that your beliefs shape where your GPS is set and that you can change your beliefs.

Where do you want to go? What does the future version of you at that destination look like? How do they feel? What do they think? What type of people do they hang around with? Why do they want to be there? What do they believe? What are the benefits of having these new beliefs? Get kinky with it.

5. Give your body what it needs

That is, the 4 Female Fundamentals.

<hr />

**Choose to be more loyal to your future self
than you are to your past self.**

So, whether it's a lottery ticket, a milkshake, Viagra, or a surprise party, our reality is impacted by the stories we believe about ourselves—but we have the power to change them. When we believe that we don't or allow them to go unchecked, our current reality is unconsciously chosen by our familiar past. We're effectively handing over control of our GPSs, which leads to us feeling lost and out of control. The moment you have control is when you realize you've been driving all along.

Chapter 6

WHERE TO NOW?

～

Living a new story.

Do you know what happens at the end of every movie? At the end of every *Queer Eye for the Straight Guy* transformation? The main character—hi, yes, that's you—realizes after all of the struggles they've been through, they had the answers all along. They knew what they needed to change, and they leaned on the support of their crazy best friend, or the cryptic message from a wise guide, and they became a different person.

The happy ending isn't the girl getting the guy (or girl); it's not winning the championship game or finally moving out of their parents' place at the age of 40. If it were, all we'd do is watch the first ten minutes and last ten minutes of a movie.

It's time to write a new story. One where we don't want to rush to the end. Instead, we get to enjoy it along the way.

THE STORIES WE'VE CARRIED

For our whole lives, as women, we've been told the story that our bodies are the problem.

That the reason for our hysteria is our uterus and removing it will cure us (hysterectomy). Told that periods are only important if you want a baby. That they're annoying, inconvenient, and painful otherwise. Told that being a woman is worse than being a man. That we shouldn't complain because others have it worse than us. That feeling fatigued, depressed, and moody is normal. That PMS and feeling our emotions makes us incapable of having a level head. Told that having a deep knowing isn't good enough and we need proof. Told that what we feel is in our head. That we're more complex than men. That women's health is an ethereal beast and we should be happy with a doctor that listens to us, even if they don't have the answers. That our stretch marks, acne, double chins, and love handles are tarnish marks, signs that we're defective and need to cover them up. If only we had a male body, it would be so much easier… Told that our intuition is to be feared, living in a world where we need to rely on health trackers to tell us something is wrong because we're so out of touch with our bodies. Where no one has ever taught us how to connect to our bodies. Where no one ever places any importance on it. Where we're bombarded with conflicting information that convinces us the answer to our problems is outside of us.

Where we've been convinced that our bodies are the problem.

LIVING A NEW STORY

I live by a new story. One where women trust their bodies. Where we live in deep connection with our bodies. Where we meet our symptoms with curiosity. Where we see our symptoms as a gift, showing us the way forward. Where we value being in connection with our bodies above all else. Where we are led by our bodies. Where we know we aren't victims of what happened in the past, but creators of what will happen in the future. Where we acknowledge our symptoms and know how to move forward. Where we have learned the language of our bodies. Where the world knows the importance of all types of healthcare and where we use our bodies as guides to know what support we need.

Where we live in a world where there's no longer "a space between" that women keep falling through. A world where we know that a diagnosis is just part of the story, not the destination. A world where we know the difference between common and normal. Where we support each other. Where we know the power of our bodies. Where practitioners remember that the body is the best doctor. Where they understand the importance of all healthcare and that it's not a rating system but a matching system. Where practitioners focus more on how to think, not what to think. Where practitioners are less concerned with what's wrong and more concerned with what happened. A world where practitioners are empowered by the body too. Where we know what type of healthcare we need and when. Where women are empowered with information and tools to know what their bodies are telling them and what to do about it. Where we realize that women's health isn't as complex as we thought it was. A world where we understand that the body is more powerful than we will ever know. A world where we're not waiting for someone or something magical to come and fix us, but where we realize we're the magic.

A world that makes the quality of our lives just as good as the quantity. A world where we're empowered with knowledge and tools to take responsibility for our own health, knowing when we need help and what type of help we need. Where women feel powerful and in control of their health. A world where we stop treating chronic illness with the same mindset as we do acute illness. Where our bodies and our womanhood aren't a burden we were given when we were born, but gifts.

A world where a diagnosis isn't the final destination but a way to better understand how we need support. Where we have access to tools for our functional and energetic health. Where we trust ourselves to know what's best for us. Where we use our bodies, not our minds, as our decision-makers.

A world where we see our bodies as the solution.

~

I was talking to my friend who spends most of his days putting cameras up people's bums and down their throats—don't worry, he's a general surgeon. He mentioned the number of people he does these tests on compared to the number of people he finds serious issues with, like bowel and stomach cancer. A common problem he has is that for the patients that have clear results on their tests, there's no real support for them. It's, "Well, you don't have cancer, growths, ulcerative colitis, or diverticulitis, so you have IBS." It's meant to be good news, which it is, but people are left in limbo. While a lot of medical professionals know this, the route for management isn't clear.

The system doesn't change unless we do.

Just like going on holidays boosts your sex drive, changing jobs gives you a whole different outlook on life, going to the gym frequently changes how you look, and holding in your truth makes you sick, your body reflects the story you continue to tell it. You have the power to change how your body feels. The anger, sadness, guilt, IBS, stretch marks, weight gain, reflux, hair loss, fatigue, endometriosis, anxiety, PCOS, fatigue, autoimmune disease, diabetes have always been gifts. Like the warning light that appears in the plane cockpit that guides the pilot to make a different decision, saving everyone on board.

Where you want your story to go is up to you. You get to rewrite it every day.

1. Listen to what your body is telling you.
2. Take care of your 4 Female Fundamentals.
3. Focus on where you want to go.
4. Let life work its magic.

It's as simple as that!

Acknowledgments

Mum and Dad

They say all you need is one person in your life to say, "You've got this," and I've been lucky enough to have two. Thank you for always meeting my curiosity with open arms and nourishing it at every twist and turn. For opening my eyes to a whole wide world, encouraging me to explore more, to create the change we wish to see, and for always being my trapeze net to come back to. I love you both tremendously.

My Family

Life has been so much sweeter having you all in it. Thank you for simultaneously being a pain in my ass and also some of the biggest loves of my life. You've helped shape some of the most important experiences of my life. I feel so lucky to have spent my life with you. I love you all.

My Chosen Family

To my Trybe, both new and old. Without your love, support, guidance, and laughter, this book never would have been possible. Thank you for being my sounding board, my emotional support, my much-needed distraction, and often my source of inspiration. I love you all.

Pixie

Thank you will never seem like enough. Thank you for helping me feel safe in my body. For showing me how to feel and helping me develop a deep, undeniable connection to my body. Thank you for having laughter in the dark. Without you, the layers would have remained armor. Thank you for reminding me that we're all the magic we've been seeking. Most of all, thank you for being my safe space when I couldn't be it for myself. It has been the greatest gift. I love you.

Nat

They say writing a book is like giving birth. While I haven't given birth to a baby yet, I couldn't have asked for a better "book midwife" than you. Thank you for your endless support. For remaining steady among my doubts. For holding me to a high standard. For pushing me to share. For meeting my vulnerability with vulnerability. For laughing with me and for helping to create something great among all of my "wonderful" grammar. I think you can add "book midwife" to your job title now.

My Patients

Your fearless hope and belief in a better way forward is a constant source of inspiration. Thank you for being brave, listening to the voice of your body over the voice of doubt, and demanding a new way forward. Without you, we would never be pushed to be better. I feel so privileged to be able to guide you towards a new, fun, and simple way to be with your body. LET'S DO THIS!

Grandma and Ancestors

Thank you for showing me the joy of caring for others and the importance of caring for myself. For being my inspiration and always guiding me forward with your cheeky and wise presence. I couldn't have done this without you. Grateful to have you by my side always...

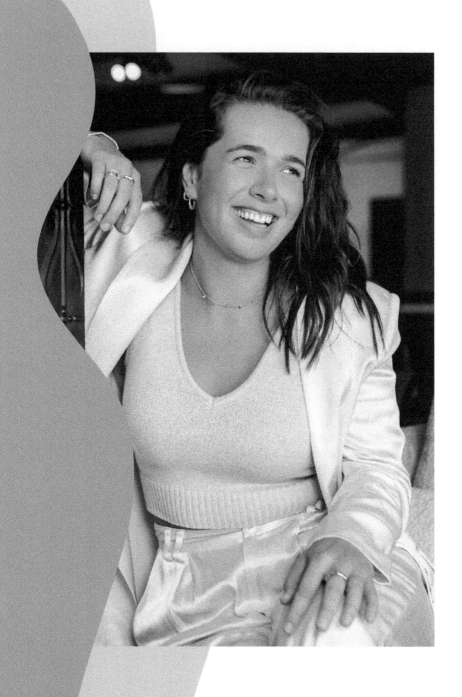

About the Author

DR. ANTHEA TODD, D.C. founded Female Fundamentals™ after observing her female patients' struggles in the complex healthcare system.

Her mission is to simplify and add fun to female healthcare.

With a background in chiropractic, a dual master's in women's health medicine and reproductive medicine, and expertise in functional medicine, functional neurology, cardiometabolic health, gastrointestinal health, immune-hormonal health, bioenergetics, and neuro-emotional technique, she's reshaping women's health.

Her goal is to empower women and professionals to see their bodies as the solution, not the problem, emphasizing that the magic we seek is within.

WWW.FEMALEFUNDAMENTALS.COM.AU

SOCIALS
Instagram: @dr.antheatodd
Youtube: femalefundamentals_4
TikTok: @femalefundamentals

Resources

You can find tools, resources, free quizzes and ways to connect with Dr. Anthea on her website, www.femalefundamentals.com.au.

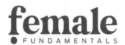

Free resources

Blogs

Quiz

Book Bonuses

Additional support

Test your Fundamentals

Membership

Practitioner Training

Endnotes

1   Maté, Gabor, and Daniel Maté. *The Myth of Normal: Trauma, Illness, and Healing in a Toxic Culture*. 2022. New York: Avery

2   Australian Institute of Health and Welfare. 2023. "Deaths in Australia." *Australian Government*. Accessed January 18, 2024. https://www.aihw.gov.au/reports/ life-expectancy-deaths/deaths-in-australia/contents/life-expectancy.

3   Heart&Stroke. n.d. "How a Healthy Heart Works." *Heart and Stroke Foundation of Canada*. Accessed January 19, 2024. https://www.heartandstroke.ca/heart-disease/ what-is-heart-disease/how-a-healthy-heart-works.

4   Advent. 2021. "How Many Breaths You Take Per Day & Why It Matters." Accessed January 19, 2024. https://adventknows.com/blog/how-many-breaths-you-take-pe r-day-why-it-matters.

5   Britannica. n.d. "Gastric Secretion." *Encyclopedia Britannica*. Accessed January 19, 2024.

6   Tseng, Julie and Jordan Poppenk. 2020. "Brain Meta-State Transitions Demarcate Thoughts Across Task Contexts Exposing the Mental Noise of Trait Neuroticism." *Nature Communications* 11 (July). doi.org/10.1038/s41467-020-17255-9.

7   Chavez-MacGregor, Mariana, Carla H. van Gils, Yvonne T. van der Schouw, Evelyn Monninkhof, Paulus A. H. van Noord, and Petra H. Peeters. 2008. "Lifetime Cumulative Number MIscof Menstrual Cycles and Serum Sex Hormone Levels in Postmenopausal Women." *Breast Cancer Research and Treatment*, 108, no. 1 (March): 101–112. doi.org/10.1007/s10549-007-9574-z.

8   Palmery, M., A. Saraceno, A. Vaiarelli, and G. Carlomagno. 2013. "Oral Contraceptives and Changes in Nutritional Requirements." *European Review for Medical and Pharmacological Sciences* 17, no. 13 (July): 1804–1813. https://pubmed.ncbi.nlm.nih. gov/23852908/; Thorp, V. J. 1980. "Effect of Oral Contraceptive Agents on Vitamin and Mineral Requirements." *Journal of the American Dietetic Association* 76, no. 6 (June): 581–584. https://pubmed.ncbi.nlm.nih.gov/7400487/.

9   World Health Organization. 2023. "Depressive Disorder (Depression)." Accessed January 19, 2024. https://www.who.int/news-room/fact-sheets/detail/depression.

10   Gaynes, Robert. 2017. "The Discovery of Penicillin—New Insights After More Than 75 Years of Clinical Use." *Emerging Infectious Diseases* 23, no. 5 (May): 849–853. https://doi.org/10.3201/eid2305.161556.

11   Australian Bureau of Statistics. 2023. "Causes of Death, Australia." Accessed January 19, 2024. https://www.abs.gov.au/statistics/health/causes-death/causes-death-australia/latest-release.

12   CDC. 2022. "PCOS (Polycystic Ovary Syndrome) and Diabetes." *U.S. Department of Health & Human Services.* Accessed January 19, 2024. https://www.cdc.gov/diabetes/basics/pcos.html.

13   Pert, Candace. 2012. *Molecules of Emotion: Why You Feel the Way You Feel.* New York: Simon & Schuster.

14   Eppinger, Ute. 2023. "Personalized Nutrition Therapy Promotes Diabetes Remission." *Medscape.* Accessed January 20, 2024. https://www.medscape.com/viewarticle/personalized-nutrition-therapy-promotes-diabetes-remission-2023a1000uj2.

15   Ainsworth, Mary D. Salter. 1969. "Object Relationships, Dependency, and Attachment: A Theoretical Review of the Infant-Mother Relationship." *Child Development* 40. 969–1026, doi.org/10.2307/1127008;

Bowlby, John. 1979. *The Making and Breaking of Affectional Bonds.* London: Tavistock.

16   Reed, Stephanie Collins, Frances R. Levin, and Suzette M. Evans. 2008. "Changes in Mood, Cognitive Performance and Appetite in the Late Luteal and Follicular Phases of the Menstrual Cycle in Women with and without PMDD (Premenstrual Dysphoric Disorder)." *Hormones and Behavior* 54, no. 1 (June): 185–93. doi.org/10.1016/j.yhbeh.2008.02.018.

17   Bhattarai, Hitesh Kumar, Shreya Shrestha, Kabita Rokka, and Rosy Shakya. 2020. "Vitamin D, Calcium, Parathyroid Hormone, and Sex Steroids in Bone Health and Effects of Aging." *Journal of Osteoporosis.* doi.org/10.1155/2020/9324505.

18   Keller, Abiola, Kristen Litzelman, Lauren E. Wisk, Torsheika Maddox, Erika Rose Cheng, Paul D. Creswell, and Whitney P. Witt. 2012. "Does the Perception That Stress Affects Health Matter? The Association with Health and Mortality." *Health Psychology* 31, no. 5 (December): 677–684. doi.org/10.1037/a0026743.

19   Porges, Stephen W. 2001. "The Polyvagal Theory: Phylogenetic Substrates of a Social Nervous System." *International Journal of Psychophysiology* 42, no. 2 (October): 123–146. doi.org/10.1016/s0167-8760(01)00162-3.

20   Segerstrom, Suzanne C. and Gregory E. Miller. 2004. "Psychological Stress and the Human Immune System: A Meta-Analytic Study of 30 Years of Inquiry." *Psychological Bulletin* 130, no. 4 (July): 601–630. doi.org/10.1037/0033-2909.130.4.601.

21   Watts, David, Dr. *Trace Elements & Other Essential Nutrients: Clinical Application of Tissue Mineral Anlaysis.* January 2015. Writers B-L-O-C-K; 7th Edition. https://interclinical.

com.au/shop/icl-wellness/trace-elements-and-other-essential-nutrients/

22   Lonigro, A., Pallini, S., Zanna, V. *et al.* Autonomic response to the Adult Attachment
      Projective in anorexia nervosa. *Eat Weight Disord* 25, 1799–1804. 2020. https://doi.
      org/10.1007/s40519-019-00792-8

23   Tsigos Constantine, Ioannis Kyrou, Eva Kassi, and George P. Chrousos. "Stress:
      Endocrine Physiology and Pathophysiology." In *Endotext [Internet]*, edited by K. R.
      Feingold, B. Anawalt, M. R. Blackman et al. South Dartmouth, MA: MDText.com,
      2020. https://www.ncbi.nlm.nih.gov/books/NBK278995/; Chrousos, George P. 2009.
      "Stress and Disorders of the Stress System." *Nature Reviews Endocrinology* 5, no. 7 (July):
      374–81. doi.org/10.1038/nrendo.2009.106.

24   Govindan, Lavanya, B. Vaishali, V. Sricharan, SP. Preejith, and Mohanasankar
      Sivaprakasam. 2022. "Impact of Posture on Heart Rate Variability of Individuals under
      Mental Workload Conditions." *2022 IEEE 10th International Conference on Serious Games and
      Applications for Health*. https://ieeexplore.ieee.org/abstract/document/9978565.

25   Domuschiev, Ivan. 2023. "What Is the Relationship between Electromagnetism and
      Cellular Metabolism in Humans?" *ResearchGate*. doi.org/10.13140/RG.2.2.33299.86565.

26   McHill, Andrew W., Edward L. Melanson, Janine Higgins, Elizabeth Connick, Thomas
      M. Moehlman, Ellen R. Stothard, and Kenneth P. Wright Jr. 2014. "Impact of
      Circadian Misalignment on Energy Metabolism During Simulated Nightshift Work."
      Proceedings of the National Academy of Sciences of the United States of America 111, no. 48
      (November): 17302–17307. doi.org/10.1073/pnas.1412021111.

27   Kruse, Jack. 2015. "Ubiquitination 25: UV Light and Poop Plants." *JackKruse.com*.
      https://jackkruse.com/ubiquitination-25-uv-light-and-poop-plants/.

28   Kruse, Jack. n.d. "Quantum Biology 4: Metabolic Syndrome." *JackKruse.com*. https://
      jackkruse.com/quantum-biology-4-metabolic-syndrome/.

29   Rashaid, Ayat Bani, Mazin Alqhazo, Dianne F. Newbury, Heba Kanaan, Mohammad
      El-khateeb, Ahmad Abukashabeh, and Feda Al-Tamimi. 2023. "Evaluation of
      Elements in Hair Samples of Children with Developmental Language Disorder
      (DLD)." *Nutritional Neuroscience* 26, no. 2 (February): 138–47. doi.org/10.1080/10284
      15X.2021.2022068.

30   Thorp, V. J. 1980. "Effect of Oral Contraceptive Agents on Vitamin and Mineral
      Requirements." *Journal of the American Dietetic Association* 76, no. 6 (June): 581–584.
      https://pubmed.ncbi.nlm.nih.gov/7400487/.

31   Segal, Thalia R. and Linda C. Giudice. 2019. "Before the Beginning: Environmental
      Exposures and Reproductive and Obstetrical Outcomes." *Fertility and Sterility* 112, no. 4
      (October): 613–621. doi.org/10.1016/j.fertnstert.2019.08.001.

32   Inchauspe, Jessie. 2022. *Glucose Revolution: The Life-Changing Power of Balancing Your Blood
      Sugar*. New York: S&S/Simon Element.

33   Felitti, Vincent J., Robert F. Anda, Dale Nordenberg, David F. Williamson, Alison M.
      Spitz, Valerie Edwards, V., Mary P. Koss, and James S. Marks. 1998. "Relationship
      of Childhood Abuse and Household Dysfunction to Many of the Leading Causes of

Death in Adults: The Adverse Childhood Experiences (ACE) Study." *American Journal of Preventive Medicine* 14, no. 4. 245–258. doi.org/10.1016/s0749-3797(98)00017-8.

34 Harris, Holly R., Friedrich Wieser, Allison F. Vitonis, Janet Rich-Edwards, Renée Boynton-Jarrett, Elizabeth R. Bertone-Johnson, and Stacey A. Missmer. 2018. "Early Life Abuse and Risk of Endometriosis." *Human Reproduction* 33, no. 9 (September): 1657–1668. doi.org/10.1093/humrep/dey248.

35 Angum, Fariha, Tahir Khan, Jasndeep Kaler, Lena Siddiqui, and Azhar Hussain. 2020. "The Prevalence of Autoimmune Disorders in Women: A Narrative Review." *Cureus* 12, no. 5. doi.org/10.7759/cureus.8094.

36 Hawkins, David R. 2015. *Transcending the Levels of Consciousness: The Stairway to Enlightenment*, 418. Carlsbad, California: Hay House Inc.

37 Nummenmaa, Lauri, Enrico Glerean, Riita Hari, and Jari K. Hietanen. 2014. "Bodily Maps of Emotions." *Proceedings of the National Academy of Sciences of the United States of America* 111, no. 2 (December): 646–651. doi.org/10.1073/pnas.1321664111.

38 Hillis, G. S., M. Woodward, A. Rodgers, C. K. Chow, Q. Li, S. Zoungas, A. Patel, R. Webster, G. D. Batty, T. Ninomiya, G. Mancia, N. R. Poulter, and J. Chalmers. 2012. "Resting Heart Rate and the Risk of Death and Cardiovascular Complications in Patients with Type 2 Diabetes Mellitus." *Diabetologia* 55, no. 5 (January) 1283–1290. doi. org/10.1007/s00125-012-2471-y.

39 Parent & Family Wellness Center. 2021. "The 90-Second Cycle of an Emotion." Accessed February 2, 2024. https://parentfamilywellness.com/blog/2021/11/19/the-90-second-cycle-of-an-emotion.

40 Alia J. Crum, William R. Corbin, Kelly D. Brownell, and Peter Salovey. 2011. "Mind over Milkshakes: Mindsets, Not Just Nutrients, Determine Ghrelin Response." *Health Psychology* 30, no. 4 (May): 424–431. doi.org/10.1037/a0023467.

41 Chavarria, Victor, João Vian, Círia Pereira, João Data-Franco, Brisa S. Fernandes, Michael Berk, and Seetal Dodd. 2017. "The Placebo and Nocebo Phenomena: Their Clinical Management and Impact on Treatment Outcomes." *Clinical Therapeutics* 39, no. 3 (March): 477–86. doi.org/10.1016/j.clinthera.2017.01.031.

42 Cavalli, Giacomo and Edith Heard. 2019. "Advances in Epigenetics Link Genetics to the Environment and Disease." *Nature* 571 (July): 489–499. doi.org/10.1038/s41586-019-1411-0.

43 Haramein, Nassim. 2019. "Unified Science Course—6.3.6 Mitochondria and Electromagnetic Signaling." *Resonance Science Foundation.* https://www.resonancescience.org/.

44 Schwartz, Richard. n.d. "Richard C. Schwartz, Ph.D. – The Founder of Internal Family Systems." *IFS Institute.* Accessed February 3, 2024. https://ifs-institute.com/about-us/richard-c-schwartz-phd.